Enlivened by Faith: Losing Weight with God's Help

By Arian T. Moore

ജ യ

Dedicated to my husband, Michael, who is the love of my life, and to, Tracy, my personal trainer, who taught me to put the Word in my workouts.

ജ യ

Editing by Evelyn Bourne, www.productivepen.com
Designed by The Fastfingers, www.thefastfingers.com
Fitness Photos by Barbara Cozart Photography, Model: Tracy Mitchell

Enlivened by Faith is published by Christian Faith and Fitness Media
ISBN: 978-0-615-66931-1
Library of Congress Control Number: 2012913793

Disclaimer: This book is not written to diagnose illness or prescribe medication for any health issues. Always consult your physician before beginning a fitness regimen, making dietary adjustments and for questions on your personal health status.
14 13 12 11 10 / 10 9 8 7 6 5 4 3 2 1

TABLE OF CONTENTS

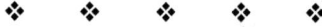

❖   ❖   ❖   ❖   ❖

ೞ ಛ

INTRODUCTION

My goal in writing this book is to show you how I lost weight using God's word. I also want to show you that He has made available all the tools that you need to accomplish this goal and maintain it. Each chapter contains a prayer for the specific topic being addressed, a tip to reiterate the topic as well as a poem to give you even more insight and motivation.

This book is not going to bore you with a slew of fitness jargon that you've heard already, but didn't understand its practicality. It's not going to give you my tips on the latest diet craze. That's not what this book is about. It's about you discovering why you have a connection to food and then showing you how, through my testimony and scriptural references, to trust God to heal those wounds.

I will to lead you through my personal battle with weight and share with you the sensible and spiritual tools that helped me to make health and fitness a part of my everyday life. Fitness cannot be an event; it has to be a lifestyle. Otherwise, after losing weight you will find yourself right back where you were. I say that in love and with the utmost tenderness. Not everyone who desires or tries to lose weight is able to maintain weight loss. In fact, most people gain back what they lost.

The National Weight Control Registry says that those who maintain weight loss are able to do so because they do the following: 1.They eat a low fat, low-calorie diet 2. They eat breakfast almost every day 3. They get about an hour of physical activity most days, often from walking 4. They monitor their weight regularly and keep track of their food intake.[1] My goal in writing this book is to help you lose weight and manage it successfully.

I want this book to inspire you. I want it to push you toward your goals—not just your weight loss goals, but all the goals that you have in life. You are more than a conqueror through Christ Jesus and you can do all things through Him.

Now go forward boldly and win!

– Arian T. Moore

---

[1] James Hill and Rena Wing. "The National Weight Control Registry," The Permanente Journal. (2003):36.

ୠ ୡ

CHAPTER 1

ୠ ୡ

In the Beginning was a word. . .

Reckless words pierce like a sword, but the tongue of the wise brings healing.

Proverbs 12:18

80 CR

From my earliest memory, I was never, "average size." As a child, I recall looking in the mirror wondering if I was adopted because my body was different than everyone else's in my family. I didn't understand why some people were fat and some were skinny. I wanted to climb out of my body and into a skinny one. I remember asking an adult to explain it to me and she said, "God makes everybody different and we are all perfect in His eyes." So why did He make me perfectly fat? That was not the answer I wanted to hear. Why were all my friends so small? Why would He want me to be the chunky kid in class? But then I figured that if God made me this way then I must be alright.

I played with the other kids and though I looked different, I felt that there was nothing wrong with me. I thought I was just as capable as the rest of them. Then I started to notice that when we played hide-and-seek I was never fast enough to make it to base. I noticed that I was out of breath riding my bike. I was always out before I even made it to second base when we played kick ball. Maybe something was wrong with me. Maybe it wasn't alright. My thoughts would later be confirmed by the comments from those around me.

"Sticks and stones may break my bones but words will never hurt me." I remember saying this time and again as a child. As I became less and less confident in myself, I received more and more insults from other people. The truth is, words really do hurt us as adults, but more importantly, as children. They left a hole in my heart that grew bigger and bigger with every attack. The banter from kids was something that I could stomach because we all teased each other, but the gut-wrenching words I'll never forget came from my very own family. I was called names like, "thunder-thighs" or "thickems."

My vision and perspective on the world around me changed. I looked at my Barbie® Doll and wondered why my stomach was not as flat as hers. I looked at magazines and television and questioned why I was not as small as those women. At the tender age of eight, I should have been thinking about school work, playing with friends and teddy bears, but instead, I worried about how different I was and how I must not be pretty since I didn't look like the images that surrounded me.

By this time I knew I was ugly. I knew that no one loved me, not even God. The words spoken to me had affected my spirit. They affected my outlook and my hope to be better. I thought I could be nothing more than what others had spoken of me. Their words had determined my destiny.

I began to eat and eat and eat. I was going through so much and I felt trapped in this dark, heavy place. I had been captured and needed rescuing. I would sneak food after dinner, not because I was hungry, but because it made me feel good. It was my friend. It comforted me and made everything else go away for the moment. Food was the perfect solace to a child who felt alone and misunderstood. It never judged me. It never talked about me and it made me feel valuable.

I remember being so greedy in school that I would go around the lunch room asking the other kids if I could have some of their food. "You want your bread?" I'd say, salivating at the plate of one of my classmates. I would be so livid with the kids that brought their own lunch to school because it always smelled and looked so much better than what the school served us. I wanted some of it and I wanted it badly. I had developed the reputation of being a beggar and it hurt—terribly, but I was hungry. I wanted food.

I wanted fried pork chops and hot dogs and cookies. My drink of choice was strawberry flavored Kool-Aid®, a drink packet mix that I loaded with white sugar. Fruits and vegetables were not high on my list of favorites—actually they weren't on there at all. My neighbor and I, and some of the other kids, would go to the candy lady (usually a retired woman that sells candy and snacks out of her home) every day. My purchase included hot fries, taffy candy and hard peanut candy. There wasn't anything better than leaving the candy lady's house with a bunch of candy—except for hearing the ice cream truck. If it was summer time that meant that the ice cream man was coming later that day and if I used all my money at the candy lady I would just run back in the house and ask my dad for some more change.

Every significant event that I recall involved food and that made it so much easier for me to fall deeper and deeper in love with it. I submerged myself in each meal. Christmas dinner was more important to me than the presents (well almost). Birthday cake and ice cream lit up my face and it is what I remember most about my birthdays. Everywhere I turned there was food. Food was always around and I enjoyed every moment of it.

Luckily for me, the children in my neighborhood still went outside to play after school every day. Although I gained weight, I never ballooned to the point where it was a risk to my health. We all rode bikes through the neighborhood; we had skates, and even raced to see who ran the fastest. I also walked to the train station after school every day with my grandma, who worked at my elementary school. One good thing about my childhood, in terms of my health, was that I stayed active.

* * * *

The Power of Words

Words have power. They have the power to create and the power to change. Proverbs 18:21 says, "The tongue has the power of life and death, and those who love it will eat its fruit." The problem is we don't realize the power we have when we speak. We destroy or bring forth fruit with the words we speak. The Message Bible, version of that same scripture says, "Words kill, words give life; they're either poison or fruit—you choose." The words that my family members said to me about my body and size killed me. They destroyed my belief that I was attractive and caused me to have an utter disgust for my body, affecting my self-esteem throughout my adulthood.

God created the world in six days by speaking it into existence. Genesis 1:3 says, "And God said, "Let there be light," and there was light." Verse six says, "And God said, "Let there be an expanse between the waters to separate water from water." He later said in Genesis 1:26, that He created us in His image and with His likeness, meaning that we are able to operate the same as the Father. Like Him, we can speak things into existence and see them manifest. By faith, we can even call things that be not as though they are.

We all operate in this power, but many times we use it to curse not bless. We speak negative things into existence all the time. In fact, this is what happened to me. I was not a fat child. I was not even obese. I had a little extra love in the mid-section. I was about eight to ten pounds heavier than the average kid my age, but let's be real here, that's smaller than today's average child. Instead of showing me how to live a healthy lifestyle, or taking walks with me, people spoke words into my life and created exactly what they spoke. They said I was fat and though I wasn't then, I eventually became fat. They called me thunder thighs and though I didn't really have them then, I surely got them later.

My Mama used to say, "If you don't have nothing nice to say, don't say nothing at all." If we all took this advice, imagine how much more we all could accomplish, how much farther we could all go? Perhaps I would not have struggled as much with my weight if those around me had spoken words of encouragement, instead of insults. As I write this, I am quite sure that the people that said these things never realized that what they said could have such an impact on my life. I am sure they don't even remember saying those things. But this shows how careless we can be with the words that we speak.

Why did I morph into what they said about me? The fact is that if you hear something long enough you begin to believe it; your heart ingests it. When you believe something, you become it. After hearing so long that I was fat, I became that. When you believe that you are the best at something, you become the best. If you believe that you are a failure, you will fail at everything that you set out to do. We cannot accomplish what we do not believe. On the other hand, what we believe becomes highly attainable for us. Your thoughts and what you believe about yourself eventually determine your destiny. Your words produce your thinking and your thinking will ultimately determine your destiny.

It was not until I became an adult that I was able to undo the damage that was done as a result of the words people spoke over me and into my life, and I accomplished this by changing my thinking. Changing your thinking can give you a different destiny; it leads you down a different road—a better road. I learned to believe what God said about me, because let's be honest here, no one's opinion but His really matters in the grand scheme of things. His words are the only ones that can save us. His words are the only words that can heal and deliver us.

What God Said About You and Me:

I am fearfully and wonderfully made.

I praise you because I am fearfully and wonderfully made; your works are wonderful, I know that full well. Psalm 139:14

He knows the number of hairs on my head.

Indeed, the very hairs of your head are all numbered. Don't be afraid; you are worth more than many sparrows. Luke 12:7

God knit me and formed me personally in my mother's womb.

For you created my inmost being; you knit me together in my mother's womb. Psalm 139:13

God loves me so much that He gave up something that He cherished just for me.

For God so loved the world that He gave His one and only Son, that whoever believes in Him shall not perish but have eternal life. John 3:16

I am His friend.

I no longer call you servants, because a servant does not know his master's business. Instead, I have called you friends, for everything that I learned from my Father I have made known to you. John 15:15

I was created in His image.

So God created man in his own image, in the image of God he created him; male and female he created them. Genesis 1:27

I allowed these words to be implanted into my heart and eventually they became heavier than the negative words that had been spoken to me. Just like their words became my thoughts and therefore my destiny as a result of hearing them over and over again, I had to hear God's words about me over and over again before they became real to me. I believed what others said so much that I came into agreement with what they said and I often spoke the same words about me that they spoke. I had to do the same thing with God's word. Those scriptures became my confessions. The Message Bible says in Proverbs 7:3 that you should etch the word of God on the chambers of your heart. The New Living Translation (NLT) says, "Write them deep within your heart." We write God's word on our hearts by meditating on it and confessing it. When we do this, we come into agreement with what God has said and come out of agreement with the negative words that were spoken over us.

Speak it

Jesus said, in Matthew 21:21 NLT, "...I tell you the truth, if you have faith and don't doubt, you can do things like this and much more. You can even say to this mountain, 'May you be lifted up and thrown into the sea,' and it will happen." Jesus is saying that if we believe and have faith we can have whatever we say. The premise is you have to believe and you will begin to believe it the more you speak it. Why? Because when you speak something or confess it over and over again you begin to see it and think it (as a man thinketh so is he..." Proverbs 23:7 KJV), eventually you have, and become what you speak.

I used this principle myself. I would say, "I will be healthy and I will lose weight." I spoke it into existence. Faith is believing something will happen even though you don't see it with your natural eyes right now (Hebrews 11:1). I believed that although I didn't see it in the mirror, I would see it soon enough. There is so much power in your mouth. If you begin to understand that you'd be more vigilant about the things you say and what you allow other people to speak into your life. Parents, be mindful of the words that you speak into the lives of your children. We walk by faith and not by sight. Your child may not be where you want them to be, but speak the thing into them that you want to see. If they are misbehaving, start thanking God that they are obedient and well-behaved. If they are involved in sin, start thanking God that they delight in righteousness. Speak by faith! Speak what you want to see, not what you see now. That's how we live by faith!

❖ ❖ ❖ ❖ ❖

TINY TIP:

Life and death is in the power of the tongue. (Proverbs 18:21) What you put in and what comes out of your mouth can lead you to either health or destruction.

ACTIVITY:

Use this trashcan to trash every negative word that has been said about you. Write those words in the trashcan. You are throwing these words away! Out of your mind and out of your life!

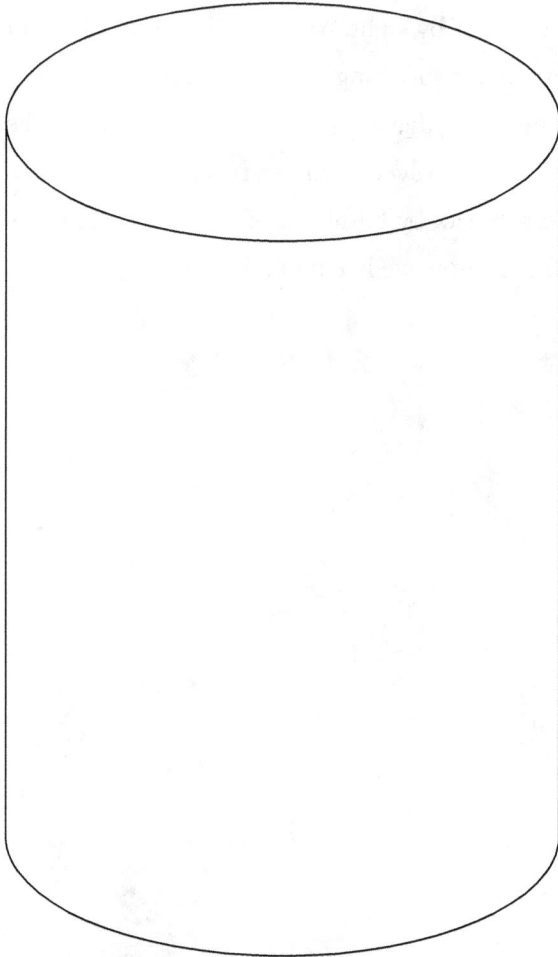

You can also take a blank piece of paper and draw a trash can for this exercise or you can simply write the words on a piece of paper and physically throw that paper away.

Use this mirror to symbolize a reflection of you. Wow! You look good! Write positive words about yourself into this mirror. As you write each word, repeat it out loud saying, "I am…"

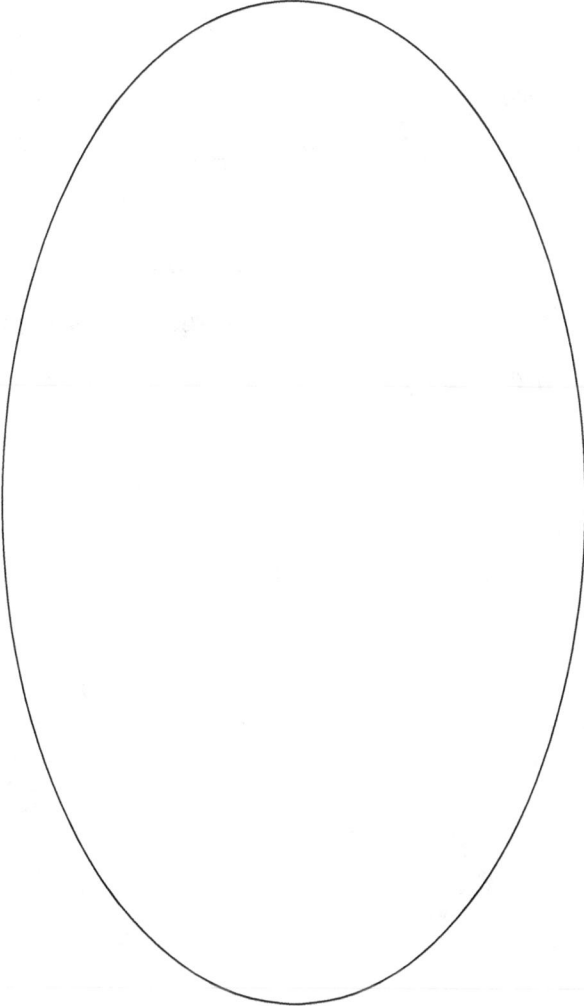

You can also use a blank piece of paper and draw an oval. Write the words in the oval (mirror) or you can use sticky notes and stick them on the mirror in your bathroom.

Prayer:

Lord I come against all the negative words that were spoken over my life. I am not ugly or fat, I am your child and your Word says that I am wonderful. Your Word says that I was created in your image and likeness and because I look like you, I bind and come against any behaviors that were established in my life as a result of those wrong words. I take on a new life and see myself through your words, not through the words of others.

In Jesus' Name,
Amen

ಕೊ ಅ

ODE TO WORDS

I will cherish the very essence of you.

Never again will I disregard your worth.

I will use you in honesty and truth,

Being loyal to your very purpose;

to inspire and birth vision.

Your nature is divine,

For with you the Earth was formed,

Oceans covered land,

And then I was created.

Never again will I use you to curse.

Never again will I listen to your misuse,

I will honor you.

I will uphold you.

One word,

God's word,

Changed my life.

ಕೊ ಅ

CHAPTER 2

A Generation of Bad Habits

Train a child in the way he should go: and when he is old, he will not turn from it.

Proverbs 22:6 KJV

၈၀ ෬

"There are kids starving in Somalia," my mom would say. "You better finish your plate." She didn't realize that she was creating a habit that would eventually lead to me being full and satisfied from a meal, but feeling like no matter what, I had to eat everything on my plate. Sometimes I just couldn't eat anymore. Sometimes I was completely stuffed, but I had to finish.

So often we do this with our children, especially those of us who work hard to keep food on the table. We somehow think that overeating is better than wasting food. Why don't we ever think of actually putting that food in some plastic containers and taking it to the local homeless shelter? If you are afraid of wasting the food, then don't waste it! Give it away! But don't force yourself to eat something you know you don't need.

When I left the nest for the first time and went to college, I incorporated those same tendencies into my eating. I never left a plate with any food on it. In fact, I often cleaned my plate with a piece of bread or a biscuit if there was any sauce left over from the meal. I carried on until I graduated and got my first place; consuming every bit of every meal no matter how full I already was.

Let's be frank here, being super full is not a pleasant feeling. It's uncomfortable to have to unbutton your pants at the dinner table because you've stuffed yourself. It's a sickening feeling. You don't know if you should lie down, sit down or stand up to get some comfort. Your stomach becomes bloated and you feel heavy. If you feel this way, imagine what your organs feel like. Imagine all that food you ate trying to travel through your intestines. Imagine how hard your digestive system is having to work.

If your fear of wasting money is what leads you to overeating think about the amount of money that you would save in healthcare costs and doctor's visits if you eat for nourishment and then stop. Or think about the amount of time and money you could save trying to lose the extra weight that you've picked up. It may seem hard to do but just throw it away, give it away or give it to the dog.

Not Knowing Better

Nutrition and exercise are subjects that have to be taught. A parent teaches their children about nutrition every time they set a plate before them. What I learned about nutrition as a child was that food was good. It made me feel good. There was nothing better than hearing the ice cream truck outside, buying my favorite ice cream and unwrapping it. That was a good feeling.

I grasped that dinner was the big meal and usually included a starch, a vegetable and a meat. My mom did a great job at always including green vegetables and she cooked dinner every night; eating out was a rare thing. She also kept fruit around the house and encouraged me to drink more water. I remember her taking me with her to walk around the track in our neighborhood. As a child I thought it was just a fun thing to do. I thought she was getting some fresh air. These things I eventually implemented into my household once I understood why she did those things. Although my mom set a pretty good example, I didn't pick up on the things she did because I did not understand their significance. (In all thy getting, get understanding. Proverbs 4:7 KJV)

I learned by observation that food was a confidant and a friend. I watched many close relatives overindulge in foods when they were lonely, stressed, depressed or simply bored. I mocked that same behavior and as an only child who was often lonely, food was my buddy. She held my hand in the dark, she danced with me and swung on the swing with me. She was an adaptable friend too. She was sugary when I needed her sweetness, salty when I felt clever and bitter when I was a bit crabby.

My grandma would tell me to eat my vegetables and drink more water, and as I look back I wish I'd listened to her then. As a child, I didn't understand why she was saying that and what she meant by it. Adults often consider themselves to be authority figures who should not have to explain themselves to children, but when you give instructions without explanation you may find that children can be curious to try the thing you told them not to do, or they do not do what you asked. Children react this way merely because they never understood and understanding is important.

The habits that I learned as a child stuck with me. In college, I gained a total of thirty pounds as a freshman. I became sick and had terrible gas. I also suffered from heart palpitations and had to undergo a stress test and EKG test at the university hospital. At only eighteen years old, I was on the road to a heart attack.

Although I walked a lot every day, because of how big my college campus was, the extra calories that I ate made losing weight impossible. It's all a numbers game. Too many people think that as long as they exercise they can eat whatever they want. This is ludicrous. You will not see results eating that way. More importantly, the goal is not simply losing weight or even looking a certain way; the overall goal is for you to live long and be strong. When you treat your body like a garbage disposal it will not be able to give you the abundant life that Jesus died for you to have. You can't accomplish the will of God for your life if you are sick and/or unhealthy.

Here is a sample of what my daily meals looked like at that time:

- Breakfast – French toast loaded with syrup, omelet and orange juice
- Lunch – Hot wings and fries
- Dinner – McChicken® sandwich and fries and an Oreo® Blizzard® milk shake with hot fudge on the top and on the bottom
- Late night snack – pizza or ramen noodles

One of my beloved dinner meals was French fries smothered in nacho cheese, ranch dressing and a ground turkey melt with extra cheese. I would top that off with a slice of chocolate cake and some punch.

Where did things go wrong? How did I get to that point? I didn't learn why we eat and what the purpose of food is. If we don't know the purpose of something we will abuse it. There is a purpose for everything. To everything there is a season, and a time for every matter or purpose under heaven. (Ecclesiastes 3:1 AMP) I thought that food was for comfort. I never understood its meaning as being for nourishment.

Could it be that the health issues we have in our families are not a result of genetic imbalances, but instead are just generations of bad eating and ignorance? I notice that high cholesterol runs in my family, but I also notice they all, for the most part, have the same eating habits. If they all changed their eating habits and became a bit more active, I believe high cholesterol would no longer be an issue.

As we raise children we set the course for their lives. They watch us and they pick up on every little thing. Psalm 127:3 says, "Sons are a heritage from the LORD, children a reward from him." God gives us these precious rewards as assignments and we are stewards over them. It is our responsibility to educate ourselves in areas where we may lack knowledge. If you have limited knowledge in the area of finances and saving money, educate yourself in that area so that you may teach your children. The same is true in the area of nutrition and exercise. Ignorance is a handicap and what they don't know will only serve as an obstacle. Don't continue to pass down bad habits, let them end with you.

* * * *

It Starts in the Womb

The stage gets set at the very beginning of our lives. Even when you become pregnant you should be eating healthier foods and exercising because those things do affect the baby. Exercise also makes labor much easier[2] and if you eat healthier you are sure not to put on as much weight. When I was pregnant, I maintained a healthy diet. Of course I gave in to some cravings (such as sending my husband out for bread sticks), but overall I stuck to a meal plan rich in whole grains, veggies, nuts and lean meats. I also worked out five times a week and in the end, I gained a total of twenty-two pounds.

My pregnancy workout was:

- A one-hour walk - Monday, Wednesday, and Friday morning
- Thirty minutes on the elliptical and 30 minutes of strength training - Tuesday and Thursday

Too often women use pregnancy as an excuse to overindulge in foods that they would otherwise not be eating in such massive quantities. The result is a woman who has gained a ton of weight and has to work twice as hard after pregnancy. My first son was born in October and by

[2]Sarah Crow, "10 Secrets to Easier Labor." www.parents.com.

January I was back to my pre-pregnancy weight. I don't say that to boast or brag, but to encourage you. Besides, it's all because of God. He gets the glory.

In addition to the practical things, my husband and I used our spiritual authority in believing for a healthy, easy pregnancy and delivery. We took communion over my pregnancy and asked others to stand in agreement with us that the pregnancy and delivery would be smooth with no complications, and that our child would be healthy and whole in every area. Remember faith without works is dead and so is works with no faith!

The first nutrition a baby needs is breast milk. Breast milk is the very reason why God gave women breasts, and nursing is mentioned a number of times in the Bible.

Scripture references:

- Song of Songs 8:1 If only you were to me like a brother, who was nursed at my mother's breasts!
- Isaiah 49:15 Can a mother forget the baby at her breast and have no compassion on the child she has borne?
- Psalm 22:9 Yet you brought me out of the womb; you made me trust in you, even at my mother's breast.

The CDC reports that breastfeeding has been shown to combat childhood obesity.[3] Breastfeeding also teaches babies to stop eating once they are full. There are a lot of free resources and organizations such as the La Leche League, dedicated to assisting moms with breast

---

[3]Centers for Disease Control, "Hospital Support for Breastfeeding: Preventing Obesity Begins in Hospitals." Cdc. gov.

feeding, however, if you are unable to breastfeed, be sure to choose a formula with as few chemicals as possible.

When baby starts eating solids, be sure to offer healthy options. Personally, I prefer pureeing fresh fruits and vegetables as opposed to the jarred foods because they contain preservatives. It's really easier than most people think. You can heat a sweet potato in the microwave, mash it and freeze it in ice trays.

I used wholesomebabyfood.momtastic.com for information on pureeing and it proved to be a great website. But if this is too time consuming for you try the organic versions of packaged baby foods. When I didn't have a chance to puree I used the Plum Organics® brand. They have different varieties of foods like mangoes and prunes.

Some foods that require less work are avocado and banana. Avocado is a great first food and all it requires is a little mashing, as is banana. As baby develops into toddler phase, continue to offer fresh veggies and fruits; frozen is also a good alternative. Most importantly, offer a variety of foods in different colors and textures.

Easy foods to puree:
- Butternut squash – bake
- Green beans – boil
- Apples – bake
- Pears - bake
- Broccoli – steam

* after cooking, puree them in a blender or food processor and freeze in an ice tray.

As your baby becomes a child and is a bit more independent, there may be different stages where he prefers some foods over others. He may only want to eat rice and apples or pasta and mangoes. Don't fret. These stages don't last forever. Let him see you eating healthy foods and he will come around. You are your child's biggest influence. Pack healthy lunches if you can and if not, teach your child how to make healthy choices at day care or school.

Taking family walks is an excellent way to demonstrate physical activity at an early age. From there, and as the children become older, you can either do family activities like exercise video games, fun workouts, or sign them up for physical activities in the community such as football, karate or soccer.

I know that you may be thinking, "Wow! That's hard work." It wasn't hard at all. When I think about the years I'm adding to my children's lives by incorporating these behaviors, it's quite effortless. Eating healthy is much easier than dealing with the hospital bills of having a child with a chronic disease.

Your child needs you! Cook healthy, live healthy, and be healthy!

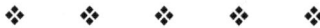

❖   ❖   ❖   ❖   ❖

TINY TIP:
Set an example for your kids by staying active! We are their role models. If they see us exercising they'll be more likely to live healthier lifestyles. Get moving and do it for your children!

Prayer:

Lord, first of all, I thank you for the effort my parents (or caregivers) made in raising me. Thank you for the food that we had to eat; that I was not starved. But Lord, I ask that you help me to eat better than what I was taught. Help me to see food as a means of nutrition and not as a form of comfort. Help me to use the bones and muscles you gave me for participating in physical activity.

I thank you for the children that you have blessed or will bless me with. I accept the assignment that you have given me to teach them and instruct them in the way they should go. Help me to show them the right way to take care of their bodies. Let me be an example for them.

Give me the desire to eat healthy and exercise. Give me tasty ideas for meals and fun ideas for activities we can do as a family. Thank you that you would touch the hearts of everyone in my household that they too might be on board for a faith filled and fit lifestyle.

In Jesus' Name,
Amen

ೲ ಛ

PLEASE TEACH ME:
A PLEA FROM YOUR CHILD

You are the hero that created me

I will forever admire you

I want to be like you

You are my parent.

Though I may not always listen

I hear everything you say

I see everything you do

You are my teacher.

Please teach me.

ೲ ಛ

ജ ൙

CHAPTER 3

ജ ൙

Wife and Mom: The Nutritionist

A wife of noble character who can find?
...she provides food for her family
... and faithful instruction is on her tongue.

Proverbs 31: 10, 15 and 26

ജ ൬

In a society where there is such a debate between women working or staying home, being a wife or mother is a tough job whether you work outside the home, work from home, or stay home. When I was working a nine to five job, I thought it was hard to find time to cook healthy meals; when I started working from home, time was not easy to come by either—especially with an infant. What I've learned is that you have to make time for the things that are important. Having your children grow up eating healthy meals is imperative to their health now and in the future.

It's easy to stop at a fast food restaurant, but it's healthier to throw some frozen broccoli in a pot with a little water and throw some sweet potatoes and some chicken in the oven. I know that many will say, "I have so much to do." Could the problem be that we are just too busy? When things matter to us we find time for them. The issue is making what you and your family eats matter to you.

Busyness, Laziness and Excuses

I think busyness is one of the reasons our country has the highest rates of childhood obesity and obesity overall. Being busy causes us to get in the drive-through line. Being busy is also the reason many of us cannot find time to exercise. We work from sun up to sun down. Psalm 39:6 NLT says, "We are merely moving shadows, and all our busy rushing ends in nothing. We heap up wealth, not knowing who will spend it." The wealth that we are working so hard to accumulate will be spent by others when we pass away. We should therefore, as the scripture goes on to say, put our hope in God and be about His business, carrying out His will. We cannot carry out God's will for our lives if the house that the Holy Spirit lives in is broken and diseased. We cannot be about His business if we are laid up in a hospital bed. How can we heal the sick when we are sick ourselves?

As we discuss busyness, we should also address the issue of laziness. Proverbs 13:4 NLT says, "Lazy people want much but get little, but those who work hard will prosper." It's amazing and somewhat frustrating to me when people ask me to help them lose weight and when I tell them how to do it they say, "I didn't know it took all of that. That's just too much." Who said it would be easy? What they are really saying is that they are not willing to do what it takes to get the job done. Without calling the people I just referenced lazy I will simply say this – the dictionary defines laziness as disinclined (reluctant or unwilling) to work. Romans 12:11 NLT says, "Never be lazy, but work hard and serve the Lord enthusiastically." If you can spend hours on Facebook in idleness and then say you don't have time to exercise—that's lazy. If you set your alarm clock for a television show (idleness) and then complain that you are too busy to cook healthy foods—that's lazy. Why? Because you are unwilling to do the work. Losing weight requires work and to see permanent results you have to be committed to doing the work for the rest of your life.

Having the right priorities is always the key. We have to have balance in our lives where we are neither too busy nor too lazy; therefore neglecting the important things in our lives. There is nothing wrong with working hard to provide for your family, however, you have to balance the other components that are critical to your life. For example: If you work all day in an office, you can take a walk for lunch. Devote weekends to your family and give God first place every day. Remember to whom much is given, much is required. Also there is nothing wrong with taking some time to relax. We all need down time. Just be sure not to neglect the other people and responsibilities that you are called to, such as living a healthy lifestyle. When we make excuses for why we can't do something, it's because we just don't want to do it. We'd rather do what we want to do and that's fine. You have a right to do whatever you want to do. Just don't complain about the weight and don't cry about the diagnosis. I apologize if that comes off as harsh but the reality is, if you want better, you have to do better. Just like a man who wants a better job has to work hard to get a better job by sending in resumes, going on interviews and maybe even going back to school, you have to work hard to have a better Body Mass Index (BMI), heart rate, blood pressure and cholesterol level.

So stop the excuses. Set aside time each day to do some activity, even if it is for ten minutes. Get moving! One trick I learned is to do some exercises like squats, sit-ups and jumping jacks during the commercials of my favorite show. To get in more movement each day I also take the stairs instead of the escalator, park the furthest away from the door to stores and walk up and down each aisle at the grocery store. And when you start exercising consistently, find ways to encourage your family to get involved.

* * * *

Making Health a Family Affair

The very first argument that my husband and I had after the, "I do's," was over food. We were actually on our honeymoon on a cruise. For those of you who haven't experienced a cruise, the food is delicious and it's all you can eat. There is food available twenty-four hours a day. My husband decided that he was hungry at midnight and wanted some pizza. That turned into an argument. The next day he ordered two dinners and two different desserts saying that the portions were not big enough. I had to do something. If he carried on this way he would end up in a hospital some day.

I had a chat with him about gluttony, explaining to him that gluttony was a sin and that by overindulging in food he was disobeying God. Ezekiel 16:49 NLT says, "Sodom's sins were pride, gluttony, and laziness, while the poor and needy suffered outside her door." Here we see the word of God define gluttony as a sin. The term gluttony is also used in the book of Proverbs. It says in Chapter 23 verses 20 and 21 of the New International Version, "Do not join those who drink too much wine or gorge themselves on meat, for drunkards and gluttons become poor. . ." When we think of poor we immediately think of finances, but you can also be poor in the spirit and in health. Overindulging in food will lead to poor health, and it can lead to financial poverty as well.

Proverbs 21:17 says, "Whoever loves pleasure will become poor; whoever loves wine and olive oil will never be rich." Again, understand that you can be both rich and poor in areas other than finances. When we spend excessive amounts of time and money chasing after pleasurable things it can lead to poverty. This means we have less time devoted to the things of the spirit, seeking and following our purpose, which should always be first place. It also means that we are spending our money frivolously and on selfish gains. We are blessed to be a blessing; we have so that we can share with others. How many homeless people could you feed if you would stop eating more than your body needs? You'd have money and food to donate to others that are not as fortunate as you are. After I explained these things to my husband, he actually understood where I was coming from.

When we returned from paradise, it was time to take on our roles as husband and wife. That's when it became clear to me that the wife sets the tone in the house. I was the cook and therefore, I was the nutritionist.

But I was ill-equipped to carry out this task. I knew nothing about nutrition. I just knew from watching my mom growing up that a wife made sure that her family had a balanced dinner every night. She never told me that, but I learned it from watching her. She made sure that we had food on the table, and for the most part we had home cooked meals. It just further proves that children are sponges and they watch what you do even when it seems that they are not listening to what you are saying.

Like me, my husband was never taught about the purpose of food. Before we met he admits to eating half of a large pizza on his own and downing six glazed doughnuts in one sitting. But he knew more about fitness than I did because he was a military fitness leader in the Navy. In fact, when we met he had a gym membership and was working out every other day. God always brings two people together that somehow complement each other.

Ironically, his eating habits were a far cry from his fitness activities and that proved to be a problem because what you eat is 80% of the battle in terms of weight loss and maintaining a healthy weight. Given that he was from New Orleans, the city known for red beans and rice, seafood Gumbo and French doughnuts, my husband didn't know much about vegetables. I remember going down there for Thanksgiving with his family and I was surprised that there were no vegetables. The only thing they had was some shredded ice berg lettuce topped with diced tomatoes. No one even touched it.

Thankfully, what I cooked is what my husband ate, and he never grumbled about me not cooking the foods that he was accustomed to eating. I look back at the beginning of our marriage and shake my head at the meals I prepared. I just didn't know any better. One of our favorite meals that I prepared was grilled Italian turkey sausages with sauteed onions and bell peppers, with melted cheese on French bread. The side item of choice was, cheese crackers. There was nothing healthy about that meal. But it was quick and easy and after working all day the last thing I wanted to do was be in a kitchen all night.

One thing that rubbed off on my husband immediately was the fact that I didn't eat any pork or beef. Now I don't say that to make anyone feel indifferent about eating meat. I still eat poultry and fish. Beef has tons of iron and when eaten on occasion can be beneficial. Pork on the other hand is not as healthy and has minimal benefits with more cons than pros. It's unquestionably a personal decision that you and your family should make, but you should stick with leaner cuts of the meats that you chose.

Because I did not buy or prepare those kinds of meats he didn't eat them. Every now and again in the early days of our marriage he would want to go to Burger King®, but after a while not eating those meats became a part of his life. He even admitted that he felt lighter on his feet; that his insides felt better.

Once I hired a trainer and learned about nutrition, of course my husband followed suit. Why? Because I am the chef and nutritionist in the house. This is such a huge responsibility that every wife and mother should understand as a part of her role. Even if your husband rejects the healthy precepts that you set into place in the home, trust God and pray for your husband. Proverbs 21:1 KJV says, "The king's heart is in the hand of the LORD, as the rivers of water: he turneth it whithersoever he will." God can change your husband's heart. Be steadfast in your prayers for him and continue to set a godly example.

1 Peter 3: 1- 2 says "Wives, in the same way be submissive to your husbands so that, if any of them do not believe the word, they may be won over without words by the behavior of their wives, when they see the purity and reverence of your lives." This scripture tells us that we can have an effect on our husbands just based on our behavior. When my husband saw me eating right, exercising and losing weight, and when he saw how much better I felt and looked he wanted to do it too. He was won over by my conduct not by my constant nagging.

If the husband is the cook of the house, the same standards can be set in place and be just as effective. In fact, as the leader of the home, you might see changes faster because your wife and children will hearken to your voice and listen to your instruction.

Eating healthy and exercising became fun to my husband and me. We started taking walks together and even running together. Eventually we both became so fit that we wanted to help other people. My husband became a personal trainer and coached other people to reach their goals. But it all started with me.

Suggestions on making fitness fun:

- Have a family race and make the prize a week off from chores
- Go for a hike together
- Go bike riding on a local nature trail
- Create an obstacle course with hula hoops, hop scotch, jump ropes and a potato sack race.

You may be in a situation where your husband or wife just likes what they like and they don't want to conform to eating healthier foods. I have a relative whose husband, although he suffers from high blood pressure and has diabetes that runs in his family, refuses to take on healthy eating habits. When she cooks baked chicken he requests that his is fried. She has to buy two different kinds of breads and milk because he doesn't like whole grain bread and low fat milk. Regardless of how well she seasons the food, he often adds extra salt.

You can't make a grown person do anything, but you can continue to set an example and pray. Prayer is a powerful thing. Too often we give up on praying for someone or something when we don't see immediate results. God is working on the hearts of people daily and in a blink of an eye that person is changed. I remember when my mom prayed and prayed for God to help her stop smoking cigarettes and one day she was just able to stop. She hasn't smoked since. What if she had stopped praying?

Children—especially teenagers—might not be so thrilled about this new way of eating that you are forcing them into. Don't make them feel coerced; make them feel like they are playing a part in making the decisions. When we cut people off from the decision making process they often rebel and whether we accept it or not, our children are individuals with their own personalities and opinions.

Here are some ways to include your kids:
- Find a healthier recipe for their favorite meal
- Flip through healthy recipes with them and ask them which ones they would like to try
- Have a cook off and give a prize to the child that makes the healthiest meal
- Bake healthier (organic, low fat and low sugar) cookies and play a family game
- Offer one day a week where the family can have one meal that they like; maybe order a pizza

One of the biggest mistakes I believe parents and teachers make is associating food with happiness. Too often celebrations and rewards include ice cream and unhealthy food options. When you reward your child with a dessert for good grades or good conduct you are causing them to associate 'good' with food. My husband and I noticed that we demonstrated this behavior. Every time we got any good news, no matter how insignificant, it was time to celebrate and that meant going out to eat (nothing healthy of course) and having a dessert. To avoid this, when your children do well in school or when they make improvements at home, try these types of rewards:

- Theme park
- Sporting event
- Extra allowance
- 15 extra awake minutes before bedtime

If you do celebrate with food, choose healthy options so that they don't correlate bad foods with good activities.

The most important thing that you can do besides setting a good example for your family is to pray for them. Our family members and friends need us to stand in the gap for them through prayer as it relates to their health and all areas of life. Lifting ourselves up in prayer should also be a daily practice. Prayer gives us power—the very same power that Jesus had and operated in—the power to remove burdens and destroy yokes.

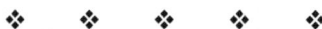

❖   ❖   ❖   ❖   ❖

TINY TIP:
Did you know that the word of God is living and active? It is according to Hebrews 4:12 AMP, which says, ". . . the Word that God speaks is alive and full of power [making it active, operative, energizing, and effective]." Sounds to me like we should be active too!

Prayer:

Lord thank you for giving me the knowledge and resources that I need to carry out the responsibility of setting a good example for my family as it relates to health. Thank you for leading me to healthy, tasty recipes and for ideas on how to get my family moving and active.

Thank you for touching the hearts of each person in my household that you would give them the desire to also honor their temple. I declare that we will glorify you with the foods that we eat and how we take care of our bodies. We will live long and strong and we will not succumb to destruction or disease. I bind obesity and every chronic disease and I declare that we are healed by the blood of Jesus.

Thank you for wisdom, for with wisdom we can do all things.

In Jesus' Name,
Amen

ॐ ଓ

WHAT'S FOR DINNER?

As much as I love you

Chicken burrito smothered in cheese,

pizza and ice cream,

I can't eat you every day.

I'll admit that when you hit my taste buds

it's like a parade;

All my fears and inhibitions go away.

A celebration in my mouth.

Yet, choosing you daily will only lead,

To weight gain

sickness

and low self-esteem.

Nope not today.

I said as I kneeled to pray.

Got people counting on me.

Refrigerator opened

What's for dinner?

ॐ ଓ

ಚಿ ಚ

CHAPTER 4

ಚಿ ಚ

Trying Everything but God

> But seek first his kingdom and his righteousness, and all these things will be given to you as well.
>
> *Matthew 6:33*

ॐ ☪

It's remarkable how society and the media have convinced us that being healthy means being a certain size. I refuse to believe that the same God that made us all different colors wanted all of us to be the same size. It just doesn't make sense to me. Even the growth and BMI (Body Mass Index) charts used by physicians have some 'cushion,' (room for varieties in different body types). Yet, when we flip through a magazine or turn on the television the men and women all look alike. The women are all identical sizes and the men all have toned abs.

As a result, instead of us wanting to lose weight to be healthy, to honor God by being good stewards, and to prevent disease, we all want to lose weight to look like the images that we see on television. And because our motives may be misplaced, we are willing to do and try just about anything to get down to that size.

Growing up around, "average-sized," people in my family, and being a bit on the chunkier side, I always felt like there was something wrong with me. That feeling was only magnified when I went to school, and even more when I was exposed to the media. I wanted to be accepted and I wanted to look like everyone else did. I did not want to be different. I decided that I would find a way to look like everyone else. Thus, began my journey of dieting.

Dieting

The first diet that I tried was a 72-hour drink diet. I was a senior in high school at the time and decided that I was tired of being called, "thick." This diet called for you to drink nothing but this juice for 72 hours and promised that you would lose at least ten pounds. I was so excited to see that my clothes were fitting more loosely. "You look good," I thought to myself staring in the mirror dressed and ready for school. Guys who hadn't paid any attention to me before seemed suddenly intrigued by me. I felt like a super star. I walked through the halls like I was walking the red carpet and peoples' teeth gleamed like flashing lights as they smiled at me walking by. I don't know if they were smiling because I looked so doggone good, or if they were laughing at me.

By the end of the day I had a pounding head ache and I became slightly dizzy. This was only day one. But I was determined to make it through to the next day because I wanted to look "normal." I wanted to look like the girls from Destiny's Child (a musical girl group that I admired) and like Britney Spears.

I lost the ten pounds, but I noticed that my skin was extra flabby. I also noticed that my face was not as clear and had become a bit darker and two-toned. My nails were extremely brittle and worst of all my breath was, for lack of a better term, "under attack." The final result was that I gained all of that weight back and then some. I know people will tell you this all the time about quick weight loss schemes, but trust me, it's not a myth.

I tried another diet similar to the one described above because I read that a few celebrities had tried it and saw dramatic results. This diet was actually created as a cleanser and the idea of the program is to purify the body and colon. Regrettably, the program has been used for weight loss purposes. It calls for cayenne pepper, water, maple syrup and lemon juice. You are also supposed to do a salt water flush in the morning (yucky) and then a laxative later in the day.

This diet, to go along with its unpleasant taste, was also an unpleasant stomach "growler." I was hungry and I had very low energy. I think I tried it a few times and each time I never made it past two days. I remember when I got my husband to do it with me. I gave him senna leaf laxative tea with two tea bags instead of one; that proved to be too much. My husband said his stomach was in knots and he was bent over. "Make it stop, make it stop," he cried, lying on the floor holding his stomach. It's actually a story that we look back on and laugh, but when you think about it, it really wasn't funny. That's the last time I ever tried that diet.

I notice that in the body of Christ, many people use fasting as a means to lose weight. I've done this before. I would go on a spiritual fast and remove certain foods from my diet for a certain time and there is nothing wrong with that. The problem with the way I was fasting was a matter of the heart. I was fasting with a greater desire to lose weight than I was to become closer to God. As Christians, our fasting should be to demonstrate discipline and a heart-felt desire to seek God; we should desire clarity and seek wisdom. Daniel said, "So I turned to the Lord God and pleaded with him in prayer and petition, in fasting, and in sackcloth and ashes." (Daniel 9:3) As a result Gabriel came to Daniel and gave him insight and understanding. It is in our fasting and praying that we hear from God and receive direction. In Acts 13:2 (NLT), we see an example of this. "One day as these men were worshiping the Lord and fasting, the Holy Spirit said, "Dedicate Barnabas and Saul for the special work to which I have called them." Despite losing a few pounds that eventually came back, I received no direction and experienced no power in my fasting. Why? Because my motives were wrong. I wanted to see results on the scale; not necessarily in my life.

Another diet that I tried was a cold cereal diet. With this diet, you eat cereal for two meals each day and then have a 'regular' meal. I ate cereal for breakfast and lunch and then had dinner. I was a sophomore in college at the time and I knew a bit more about activity so I borrowed a weight loss DVD from a friend of mine and started doing that each day. I saw results within two weeks. "Your neck looks smaller," my roommate said. "I can tell that you've been working out." That's exactly what I needed to hear. Unfortunately, I became tired of cereal. My taste buds became so bored with it that I just couldn't stick to the diet. So the weight came back.

Lastly, I tried diet pills. I tried a much publicized weight loss pill when I had hired a trainer because I wanted to see results fast (overnight). I figured the pill would be a great addition to eating and exercise. This pill scared me to death almost literally. It sped up my heart rate so much so that I could feel my heart beating through my chest. I thought I was going to die. I learned later that the pill contained ephedra, which was later taken out of stores and banned by the FDA as it was said to pose "unreasonable risk of illness or injury."

I tried a green tea pill that was supposed to speed up your metabolism. I came across it in the grocery store and just couldn't resist. I didn't see the results from that one after a month so I just stopped taking them.

I wanted to try the Jenny Craig® diet program so badly, but I could not afford the meals. I do know lots of people who tried Jenny Craig® and the Nutri System® diet program and they all had success. So yes, these programs do work, but you still have to change your thinking about food to have long-term success on such programs. What's the use in losing weight this year only to gain back double next year? For my friends who tried the aforementioned programs, they lost weight, but the minute they got off the designed meal plan, they gained the weight back. They did not know how to eat regular foods outside of what was prepared for them through the programs. The programs limit your caloric intake and that will help you lose weight, but if you are unable to translate that same caloric limitation into your lifestyle, you will not be among those who lose weight permanently.

I also tried a grapefruit pill diet. It was also supposed to speed up my metabolism, but again I saw no results. Do you see a trend here? First of all I was depending on a pill to do all the work while I continued on in the same behavior. I was not exercising and I made no changes to my eating habits. This is what we call being lazy, wanting results, but also being unwilling to do the work to see the results. There is no such thing as a magic pill. Even if there were such a thing why would you want it?

Some of those diet pills can do more harm than good. For example, taking performance enhancements such as creatine as a supplement can affect the kidney functioning properly [4] and weight loss pills like Ali, are now being said to affect the liver. [5] This is why you always want to pay attention to the ingredients in your food and anything that you put in your mouth. It should have natural ingredients that you can pronounce. You have to keep in mind that the ultimate goal is to be healthy, not to just look a certain way. You'd be flabbergasted by the number of "small" people that die from heart attacks every day. Because being small does not inevitably mean healthy, the same way that not being, "average," does not equate to unhealthiness.

---

[4] Medline Plus. U.S. National Library of Medicine. National Institutes of Health, "Creatine." Nlm.nih.gov

[5] Lara Salahi, "Weight Loss Drugs: Public Citizen Calls for Ban on Alli, Xenical." *ABCNews.* April 14, 2011. Abcnewsgo.com

Are You Healthy?

What do we mean when we say be healthy? From a natural standpoint, being healthy means that you are in good physical condition. It means that your numbers are good (blood pressure, cholesterol, and blood sugar). From a spiritual perspective, being healthy means that we have a relationship with God in which we honor Him and seek Him, and that we allow His word to be the final authority over our lives. Proverbs 4:20-22 says, "My son, pay attention to what I say; turn your ear to my words. Do not let them out of your sight, keep them within your heart; for they are life to those who find them and health to one's whole body." God's word is our source for everything and in this scripture we particularly see that His word is our source for health. This is why we must turn to the word and not to diet fads and pills.

Being healthy also means that we have a sound mind; that we are not burdened with mental confusion, tormented with negative and unhealthy thoughts and living our lives according to fear. Often times these very characteristics are what lead us to addictions and dependencies. 2 Timothy 1:7 KJV says, "For God hath not given us the spirit of fear; but of power, and of love, and of a sound mind." Moreover, we are told that we have been given the very mind of Christ. (1 Corinthians 2:16) Thus, having a sound mind is something that we have been given by God, just like we have been given Jesus, but we must accept those gifts. Receive and accept a sound mind today knowing that you don't have to be tormented by your past or burdened with evil thoughts.

Make this declaration:

I, _____, declare that in the name of Jesus I am no longer confused and tormented. I no longer walk in fear, making every decision based on the fear of the unknown. Instead, I walk in perfect love, for perfect love, which is the love of Christ, drives out all fear. I continue to renew my mind with the word of God, taking on His thoughts in exchange for my own.

Scripture reference: 1 John 4:18 There is no fear in love. But perfect love drives out fear, because fear has to do with punishment. The one who fears is not made perfect in love.

* * * *

Quick Results Don't Last

It's sad that we live in such a microwave society. We want everything fast with no work. There is a process for everything and in most instances when we take the short route; we end right back where we started. Isn't it more important to arrive at the destination than it is to get there faster? But because we want everything now with minimal discomfort, we are willing to spend money on every new pill or contraption to lose weight. This is why quick weight loss programs are so enticing to us, because they are advertised as if they require little work from us. We are made to believe that the pill or the program is going to do the majority of the work for us. Disappointingly, we don't read the small print at the bottom of the commercial that says, "These results are not typical" and "Results occurred with pill in addition to diet and exercise."

At the end of the day you are wasting money if you expect for some external object to do what you need to do internally. You have to make a decision. Are you going to live healthy or are you going to stay the same? Trying diet after diet has kept you the same so far.

Dieting does not work. If it did the obesity rates in America would not be as high as they are with over 70% of our population overweight or obese. Americans spend over $40 billion dollars a year on weight loss products and programs. Yet, every year the rates of chronic disease and obesity continue to increase. In 2009, Eric Schlosser said in his book, *Fast Food Nation: The Dark Side of the All-American Meal,* that Americans spend over $110 billion on fast food.[6] As a nation we spend twice as much on fast food as we do on weight loss products. Therefore, the programs don't work.

One reason these fad diets don't work is because we are more concerned with looking a certain way than we are with being healthy. The problem with being size obsessed is that we are never happy. That's right. I said it. You will never be happy with your size if all you are aiming to do is get down to a certain size. I know it because I went through it. When I went from a size fourteen to an eight, a size eight wasn't good enough anymore. I wanted to be a six. Then a size six wasn't good enough, so I wanted to be a four. Then a size four wasn't small enough. I wanted to be a two. When I got down to a size two guess what? That still was not good enough. I still wanted more; I wanted even smaller thighs. My arms were not as toned as they could be. My butt wasn't as tight as I wanted it to be.

For some who haven't started the weight loss journey this may sound ridiculous. But when you are chasing a number on a scale or a specific jean size this is what can happen. If your goal is to lose twenty pounds before your 50th birthday, once you get to twenty, you might say, "maybe five more." It's just like the woman going in for plastic surgery. After one procedure, she finds something else she doesn't like and then later something else. Years later she's had double digit surgeries and still is unhappy with her image.

---

[6] Eric Schlosser, *Fast Food Nation: The Darks Side of the All-American Meal.* New York, NY: Harper Collins, 2009.

Why are we like this? Because we are chasing after numbers, false images and sizes; tangible and temporal things that mean nothing in the grand scheme of things. It's how society has trained us to be—always wanting more, bigger and better. You finally get a job and a house and a year later that job and house aren't good enough. You want bigger; you want the latest trend. It's called lust. 1 John 2:16 NLT says, "For the world offers only a craving for physical pleasure, a craving for everything we see, and pride in our achievements and possessions. These are not from the Father, but are from this world."

We are supposed to be chasing after God and things of God. We have to put God first in everything that we do. In fact, our objective for losing weight shouldn't be for selfish reasons (being a certain size), but so we can be healthy vessels, ready and able to carry out any work He requires of us.

Another reason these weight loss fad diets don't work is because they don't help you to discover the reason you are overeating. Food in and of itself is not the issue. I remember watching *The Oprah Winfrey Show* once and she talked about how she discovered her connection to food. She understood that because of the trauma she experienced in her life, she had become dependent on food and even called herself a food addict. For many of us this is the case. Like a drug, food numbs the pain; it makes it all better.

I realized that I depended on food to make me feel better. As I discussed previously, food became my friend. I ran to it whenever I was depressed or lonely. Unlike people, food never hurt me, it never judged me and it never made me feel inferior. But while it deadens that pain momentarily, like any drug, the side effects are damaging and often hard to undo, especially because most of us desire unhealthy foods when it comes to comfort.

Ask yourself, "Why do I overeat?" Is it because of something that happened to you as a child? Is it because of abuse or divorce or even depression? Be honest with yourself and discover where you are. It may take some time and you may even have to ask the people around you that love you for help. Ask God to reveal it to you. You can seek the help of a counselor, minister or weight loss coach as well.

Fill in the blank below.

I overeat because _____

_____. Once you discover your connection to food, it's easier to begin the healing process, and that process includes you giving over your past and your hurts to God, letting Him fill those voids. When you call on Him to comfort you, you will no longer need the comfort of food. But when we run to every new diet fad; no carbohydrates, all carbohydrates, weight loss shakes and smoothies, we are putting ourselves on a never ending spinning wheel of disappointment and frustration.

* * * *

I hired a trainer at my church gym because the prices were much more sensible than the local gyms. God sent me to the right person at the right time in my life. My trainer was an advocate for, "putting the word of God in your workout." We prayed before each session and at the end of every session. We even incorporated scripture into our workouts, and I believe that this is the reason I was able to lose weight and maintain the weight loss.

As Christians, we are supposed to seek God in all that we do (Matthew 6:33). He alone is our source for everything. Because we live in this world, it's easy for us to depend on other things instead of leaning and depending on God. Before praying and asking God to help us lose weight, we grab a weight loss pill expecting it to be the answer. God and His word should always be the answer for the Christian.

For some it may seem silly or even radical to pray about weight loss, to seek God for help in the area of healthy eating and to pray for strength and wisdom when we exercise. If God said seek Him in all things, I believe that's exactly what He meant. Our dependency on God is not to make us feel powerless or out of control, but it is to relieve us of the stress, pressure and worry that comes with trying to do things in our own strength. We weren't designed to operate this way.

When we do things the way the world does things we get the same results they get. Our results should be unchangeable—not fleeting or temporal—however, these are the results we get when we do things like the world does things.

I often compare a weight loss journey to defeating a giant because that huge number on the scale often seems impossible to change. We are taught how to defeat giants in God's word. Notice that when David defeated Goliath his confidence was not in his ability, but in God's ability. David said, in 1 Samuel 17:46, "This day the Lord will deliver you into my hands, and I'll strike you down and cut off your head." Perhaps David would have been killed had he approached Goliath with the mindset of doing it all on his own. Yet David defeated the giant because he trusted God and depended on Him. You will defeat your giants the same way. If there is anything that seems too hard for you to handle, any battle that's too tough for you to fight remember that you never fight alone. The battle is the Lord's!

TINY TIP:
Do you think the weight is the issue? You think wrongly. Find the issue with food; lose the weight!

Prayer:

Lord I want to thank you for helping me to understand that I should seek you first in everything I do—even in my attempts to live a healthier lifestyle. I pray that you would lead me and guide me in this area. Help me to depend on you for help and the Holy Spirit for comfort.

Lord, forgive me for misusing my body for so long. Help me to forgive anyone who has hurt me and I forgive myself for any mistakes that I have made. Now Lord, I move past those things. I will no longer allow them to consume me and cause me to seek the comfort of food to numb my pain. I declare that I am set free and delivered.

I will not allow myself to be burdened with wanting to be a certain weight or size. My goal is to be healthy. Help me to keep health at the forefront of my thoughts. Help me to acknowledge you as I continue on this journey.

In Jesus' Name,
Amen

ॐ ☙

WHAT ELSE YOU GOT?

Tried the pills,

bought the DVD

Anything else you got?

Something has to work for me.

Tried the shakes,

Bought the treadmill,

But no changes on the scale.

How can that be?

All I want to do is lose this gut,

Oh and, maybe I can tighten my butt.

What else you got?

I'm willing…

NOT!

ॐ ☙

සෙ ෴ ඥ

CHAPTER 5

සෙ ෴ ඥ

There's a War Going On

Put on the full armor of God, so that you can take your stand against the devil's schemes.

Ephesians 6:11

₰ ᘓ

Sometimes believers can feel lost and left feeling hopeless when they are faced with uncomfortable situations, or battles, if you will. In fact, many of us give up or give in before we see the manifestations of God. We must first recognize that any internal struggle or stronghold is a spiritual fight and not a natural one. That's why it can't be won with pills and weight loss potions. It can only be won with the word of God (faith in God's word and total dependence on Him) and healthy behavior (actions).

The enemy uses our feelings of inferiority, our hurts and pains to entice us to turn to sin, which eventually distracts us away from God. Gluttony is in fact a sin and sin leads to condemnation and separation from the Father. Isaiah 59:2 says, "But your iniquities have separated you from your God; And your sins have hidden His face from you, So that He will not hear." This is why it is so important for us to get up from sin when we fall.

Notice that I didn't stay on the topic of sin or put too much emphasis on it. I don't want to beat you over the head because that didn't prove to be effective for me. I've been to churches where sin is the entire focus of every sermon, every Sunday. Instead of being motivated to change, I would feel unworthy and overwhelmed with flaws to work on. A few years ago I had a situation where I ate a huge dinner and was offered a slice of cake. Not only did I eat one slice, I had two slices and some ice cream. I felt horrible, inside and out, but I repented and kept going on my journey towards a healthy lifestyle. I have friends and relatives who give up after a situation like the one I just described, believing that they just can't do better or that the struggle is too hard to overcome. Neither is true and both are simply tricks of the enemy. Ask for forgiveness, turn away from the behavior and press forward.

Not only does Satan want to distract us, but ultimately, he wants to destroy us. John 10:10 KJV says, "The thief cometh not, but for to steal, and to kill, and to destroy…" He wants to steal your health by drawing you closer to food and further away from God. He wants you to seek food as your comforter. Don't you find it fascinating that when we crave foods we never long for the foods that are healthy for us? Don't you find it even more interesting that heart disease is the number one killer of Americans? This means that in most cases, our lack of activity and poor eating habits are killing us. Food cannot stand in the way of us carrying out God's will.

Satan, Food and Temptation

I have come to believe that Satan has a thing about food and temptation. The very first act of tempting that we see in the Bible that resulted in the Fall of Man had to do with Satan tempting Adam and Eve with a fruit (Genesis 3). Satan also tempted Jesus with food in Matthew 4:3. "The tempter came to him and said, "If you are the Son of God, tell these stones to become bread." This was tempting for Jesus because he was on a forty day fast. I don't know about you, but after fasting for one day a piece of bread is tempting. I can only imagine how tempting it was after forty days. But look at how Jesus responded to Satan's temptation in verse four. "And Jesus answered him, saying, "It is written: 'Man does not live on bread alone, but on every word that comes from the mouth of God.'"

This is how you can respond when he tempts you with food. You can let the enemy know that you don't live off of bread; you live off of the word of God. As you say that, you help to change your thinking about why you are eating food in the first place. When you change your thinking, you change your life. Remember, as a man thinketh in his heart so is he. If you think you can't live without junk food, you can't. If you think you can't lose weight, you won't. When you believe and think positively, you will see the affirmative results.

By responding with the word of God you put yourself in a position to win the battle. Why? Because you demonstrate that your strength is in God and His word, not in your own ability. Ephesians 6:13 NLT says, "Therefore, put on every piece of God's armor so you will be able to resist the enemy in the time of evil. Then after the battle you will still be standing firm." His armor is His word. You will be standing firm because you stood on the solid rock. Just like David did.

What is temptation in the area of eating and exercising? When you just ate lunch, are completely satisfied and a co-worker orders a pizza and offers you a slice, that's temptation. When you've finished dinner and for no other reason than habit, you are craving something sweet so bad that you're on the verge of jumping in the car and heading to the doughnut shop, that's temptation. When you've had one slice of cake and it was so good that you are contemplating having another piece, that's temptation. For others temptation might be hitting the snooze button on your alarm clock when it goes off in the morning attempting to wake you up to work out. Satan tempts us to lead us off the path of righteousness and onto a path of destruction.

Win it in the Spirit

If you talk to any addict regardless of their drug of choice, they all have one thing in common, and you'll discover it if you dig deeply enough. Most of them have dealt with abuse, neglect, ridicule, disappointment and/or depression. All of us have a dependence on something, and I say all because there is not a single person on this planet that has not dealt with the feelings that I mention above. We all self medicate to combat those feelings in one way or another. Some people prefer food while others choose cocaine. One person opts for shopping while another may choose sex. Regardless of the drug, you must first understand that this battle is not yours to fight. In The Message Bible, Deuteronomy 20:2-3 says, "Don't fear. Don't hesitate. Don't panic. God, your God, is right there with you, fighting with you against your enemies, fighting to win."

This is a spiritual battle and it is therefore won in the spirit. Ephesians 6:12 says, "For our struggle is not against flesh and blood, but against the rulers, against the authorities, against the powers of this dark world and against the spiritual forces of evil in the heavenly realms." It's not the food, it's the enemy. But you have dominion over him and he can only operate in the authority that you give him. Luke 10:19 NKJV says, "Behold, I give you the authority to trample on serpents and scorpions, and over all the power of the enemy, and nothing shall by any means hurt you." Walk in the authority that you have been given and identify with your place. You have power over him, not the other way around.

We've been left with promises such as healing, prosperity and protection. When a battle occurs, we look at our promises and let that word determine how we are going to come out. Our faith and focus should be on God and His word not our circumstances. One of my favorite promises is found in John 15:7 in The Amplified Bible, which says, "If you live in Me [abide vitally united to Me] and My words remain in you and continue to live in your hearts, ask whatever you will, and it shall be done for you." This means that if I continue in His word, I can ask for anything, even help with losing weight, and it will be done for me (as long as I ask with right motives- James 4:3 and a forgiving heart – Mark 11:25). We have to accept the Word of God as finality in our lives.

If the Bible says we are healed, no matter what the doctor says, we know that we are healed. Healing is not just needed or meant for physical sickness, it is also available for emotional ailments. You have a right to be healed and delivered from your dependence on food. Isaiah 53:5 says, "But he was pierced for our transgressions, he was crushed for our iniquities; the punishment that brought us peace was on him, and by his wounds we are healed." Not only are you healed from your dependence on food, but you are healed from the wounds that caused this dependency. That's right! You are healed from the wounds of abuse and rejection, from the wounds of lies and betrayal. You are healed! I am healed! Like you, I have dealt with a lot of trauma in my life. People hurt me, abused me, neglected and rejected me, but I am healed today because of the price Jesus paid.

There has to be a determination within you that says no matter what, I'm going to keep going. I won't give up. I won't stop and I won't quit. You owe it to yourself to be healthy and you owe it to Jesus because of the huge price he paid, to honor him by caring for your body. When I think of resolve I think of Nehemiah. He was determined to rebuild the walls of Jerusalem despite the ridicule that he faced (Nehemiah 2:19-20). I also think about the Israelites marching around the city of Jericho seven times until the walls fell down (Joshua 6:15-16). I can only imagine that people laughed at them. But they persevered because they saw the bigger picture, and because they were unwavering.

When I decided to live healthy I faced scorn and even shame. People called me, "health freak," or made snide comments like, "Oh I forgot you don't eat anything." By this time I had grown so convinced of God's word that people's remarks didn't move me. You must also get to that place where you are unmovable and unshaken; like a tree planted. When you can't be beaten by Satan and you overcome bondage to people, you have already won the battle.

Something has to be said about the way we let people affect the way we view ourselves. We talked about this in Chapter 1 when we dealt with the words that people speak about us and into our lives. But it's also critical that we not allow people's opinions to affect the decisions we make for our lives. Just because your whole family eats a certain way, don't feel that you have to compromise in order to please them. Galatians 1:10 NLT says, "Obviously, I'm not trying to win the approval of people, but of God. If pleasing people were my goal, I would not be Christ's servant." When I was a people pleaser (I use the word, "was," because those days are long gone), I was so unhappy. I was too busy trying to please people and therefore, I was not as busy trying to please God or do what was best for me. You have to be your own advocate. You would be surprised to know that the same people that ridiculed me eventually made changes and even came to me for advice and suggestions.

Lastly, we are taught through God's word that we should cast our cares on Him. 1 Peter 5:7 KJV says, "Casting all your care upon him; for he careth for you." Whatever it is that you went through in the past, give it over to God. Don't live with it anymore. Satan wants you to stay focused on you and to keep you looking back, that way you will never progress to the next level. Press towards the mark. Philippians 3:13-14 KJV says, ". . .forgetting those things which are behind, and reaching forth unto those things which are before, I press toward the mark for the prize of the high calling of God in Christ Jesus." Forget your past and let it go. Your past will no longer impinge on your future.

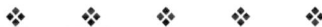

❖   ❖   ❖   ❖   ❖

TINY TIP:
Run to God! Run from evil! Your body will grow with health; your very bones will vibrate with life! (Proverbs 3:7 Message Bible)

Prayer:

I declare in the name of Jesus that I am healed by his stripes from every hurt and every pain and everything from my past. I declare that I am healed from any sickness or disease that doctors have spoken over me. I thank you for your Word and for your son Jesus, who bore my sins and my diseases and as a result I am healed, delivered and set free. I let go of my past and I cast all of those cares on you Lord.

I declare that the enemy has no victory and no authority over my life. I bind his every scheme and every obstacle that he would put in my way. I will not be defeated because you are my shield. Thank you for the victory!

In Jesus' Name,
Amen

ೞ ಚ

THE CHAMP IS HERE

Stepped in the ring afraid,

The opponent in the other corner's a bit bigger than me,

I looked to my left,

Then to my right,

I chuckled and grinned,

I will win this fight.

He's here with me,

And will fight the battle,

Doesn't matter how big the competition is,

Or what weapons he brought,

The fight is fixed cause…

The champ is here.

ೞ ಚ

CHAPTER 6

Renewing Your Mind

Do not conform to the pattern of this world, but be transformed by the renewing of your mind.

Romans 12:2

ॐ ෧

Being born again does not mean that we physically go through
the birthing process a second time. It means that we become
new creatures and that newness is demonstrated in our novel way of
thinking, our fresh outlook and the new way in which we go about
things. We develop an unsullied mindset by hearing the word of God
and letting that word change our view. Any activities that we participated
in before that do not line up with the word such as sexual immorality,
lust or stealing, we begin the process of eliminating those things from
our lives.

This development is called renewing your mind. We are being
renewed; made new by becoming like God and taking on His mindset and
His way of doing things as explained in His word. I remember thinking
that we became renewed the minute we said the prayer of salvation
or accepted Jesus into our hearts. Then I examined that scripture a bit
more carefully (Romans 12:2), and what I discovered was we are to be
transformed by the renewing of our minds. The –ing on the word renew
demonstrates that this is not a onetime event, but an on-going process.
2 Corinthians 4:16 says, ". . . Though outwardly we are wasting away, yet
inwardly we are being renewed day by day." We are renewed daily.

How does being renewed apply to weight loss and healthy living?
Well, as I expressed earlier, most of us overeat because we have a
connection to food—a food addiction. To overcome any type of sin,
the first place we must go is to God's word. We find the scriptures on
deliverance and scriptures that pertain to our particular issue and we
take on those thoughts as we meditate on those scriptures. But once we

reach our goals, we don't stop meditating on the word that helped get us there. We keep renewing our minds so that we never go back to that place.

As I stated before, I hired a trainer at my church (Tracy) and she told me to find a scripture that motivated me. Then she said to take a multivitamin and to meditate on that scripture each day. The scripture I chose was 1 Corinthians 9:27 which says, "No, I beat my body and make it my slave so that after I have preached to others, I myself will not be disqualified for the prize." I chose this scripture because I was very adamant about making better lifestyle choices. I made that known to those around me, but I could not be preaching to others if I could not make the same changes I was encouraging them to make.

As I meditated on that scripture I became increasingly motivated to live better and eat better. As I beat my body through exercise, I became so pumped up knowing that losing weight was not just about me, it was about my family and others that God would call me to. The New Living Translation of that scripture says, "I discipline my body like an athlete, training it to do what it should. Otherwise, I fear that after preaching to others I myself might be disqualified—[a hypocrite]." I was saying that I bring my body under my control and I am no longer allowing it to control me.

Another thing I did was meditate on teachings that concerned temperance and self-control. "Faith cometh by hearing." (Romans 10:17 KJV). In order for me to get the faith I need to carry out this task and the faith to believe God is able to help me to reach my goals, I have to hear the Word of God. I listened to my CD's every day, over and over again.

Perhaps the scripture that motivated me does not stimulate you. Maybe that's not where you are. That's understandable. Read Romans

12:1. It says, "Therefore, I urge you, brothers, in view of God's mercy, to offer your bodies as living sacrifices, holy and pleasing to God—this is your spiritual act of worship." Did you get that? When you honor God with your body this is an act of worship towards Him. The King James Version of this scripture says that we should present our bodies as a living sacrifice and that this is our reasonable service. Exercising is your reasonable service to God. When you take care of His temple, you honor Him.

When I got this revelation every workout session became personal time with God and worship towards Him. There were times when I cried on the elliptical machine, praising God for how good He had been to me. There were times when the Holy Spirit just came over me while I jogged on the treadmill and all I could do was pray. I'd close my eyes and see myself in the presence of God. There was no one there but Him and me. His presence covered me like a blanket and in his warmth, all of my inhibitions left. I'm not trying to be too deep or super-spiritual. I'm just sharing with you what helped me. If you want to join me there, be open-minded to all God can do and don't limit Him based on your own understanding. He's a limitless God!

I also sowed a financial seed for what I was believing for. Again, I am not telling you what to do; I'm simply unfolding the actions that I took. I was taught that God honors sacrifice and at that time in my life, the seed that I sowed was an enormous sacrifice. I wrote on the back of my offering envelope a prayer asking God to help me to lose weight so I could be in the best of health and honor Him with my body. By doing so, I further acknowledged that I was leaning and depending on Him, not my own strength, not even my personal trainer.

To sum it up, here's what you need to do first: find a scripture and meditate on it so much that it becomes real to you—so that you have memorized it and it becomes a part of you. That scripture will begin to grow and take root in your spirit and it will help you to develop self-control in the area of your eating habits and develop consistency in your workout.

Other Motivational Scriptures

Do you not know that your bodies are temples of the Holy Spirit, who is in you, whom you have received from God? You are not your own; you were bought at a price. Therefore honor God with your bodies. 1 Corinthians 6:19-20

Explanation for motivation – You honor God with your body by not subjecting it to anything that would harm it or cause it pain. In other words, don't treat your body like a garbage disposal!

For physical training is of some value, but godliness has value for all things, holding promise for both the present life and the life to come. 1 Timothy 4:8

Explanation for motivation – Physical training and exercise is important, but even more important than that is seeking after the things of God.

* * * * *

Renewing Your Mind on Food

I have to have my ice cream (now it's almond ice cream as I've become extremely lactose intolerant). All of us have a, "must have," food. For my best friend it's cheese and for my husband it's pizza. You must first confess that you don't have to have anything. You just want it. It's important that you set your priorities in order and understand the difference between wants and needs. Saying that you have to have something categorizes it as a need. I will not tell you that you can never have the foods that you love again. That's an unrealistic way to live, and for many it's simply impractical. What I will suggest is that you find a way to incorporate the foods that you love into your meal plan in a prudent way by: 1. finding a healthier way to prepare those foods or, 2. having them only on occasion—perhaps once a week. Ultimately, you clearly have to change the way you view food and its purpose.

After I began the course of renewing my mind in the spirit, I also had to renovate my mind in the natural as it related to what I thought about food. I had to recondition my mind in terms of taste and the very purpose of food. I had to change the way I viewed fruits and vegetables and even water. I had to educate myself on what to eat and how to prepare it in a way that would be beneficial to my body.

I asked my trainer lots of questions about food, calories and fat. The first thing she asked me to do was to keep a food diary for a week. She asked me to write down everything I put into my mouth, even peppermint or gum. After the week was up she would take a look at the diary and let me know what changes I needed to make. Here is what my first food diary entries looked like:

Day 1 of Week 1:

- Breakfast – One bowl of sweet, fruity cereal with whole milk and a tall glass of orange juice
- Lunch – Baked potato with cheese, turkey bacon, fried chicken and lemonade

- Dinner – Two slices of pizza with fruit punch
- Dessert – Brownie sundae

Day 2 of Week 1:
- Breakfast – Two bowls of sweet, fruity cereal
- Lunch – Turkey chili loaded with sour cream and cheese and lemonade
- Dinner – Pasta made with ground beef and cheese and orange juice
- Dessert – Chocolate candy

Because there was no variety in what I ate, every day looked about the same. When I turned it in to my trainer, she told me that I was eating too much food and that I needed to eat more fruits, vegetables and whole grains. She said, "You have to drink more water; your body needs it to function." What did she mean by too much food? I thought we just eat until we get full. She told me that the average person requires about 2,000 calories per day but when we eat more than that and incorporate no physical activity, we gain weight. Being a writer, not a mathematician, I became frustrated. "Don't get into numbers," she said. "Just remember that we eat to live, we don't live to eat!"

When I initially started training with Tracy my goal was to lose ten pounds by my birthday (wrong motives). I purchased ten sessions of training and got two free. By session five, I was not seeing the results I wanted to see. I thought the weight was just supposed to fall off— at least that's the impression we are given by weight loss commercials. Something had to be wrong, right?

Remember that what you are eating always outweighs the work you do in a gym. I was not seeing results because I had some work to do on my eating habits. I remember drawing a picture of my body for Tracy and showing her where I wanted to lose each pound. Reluctantly she told me, "Look, losing weight is all about taking in less calories than what you are putting out." She went on to tell me that one pound was equivalent to 3500 calories and to lose weight I needed to eat less than that each day. I later understood the reason she was reluctant to share the notion of calorie counting with me. She knew that calorie counting and even checking the scale on a daily basis would result in obsessive behavior.

The idea was to eat in a levelheaded way; counting calories can get you hung up on the numbers and away from the nutrition and benefits of healthy food. (We'll talk about this more in the next chapter). Because I was perturbed, she asked to take a look at my food diary. While I had made some changes, I still had more changes to make. Here is what my Day 1 of Week 3 looked like (I was training two days per week and on the other three days I did cardio and strength training).

Day 1 of Week 3:

- Breakfast: One nutrition shake and one granola bar
- Lunch: Grilled chicken, baked potato with low fat butter and a salad
- Dinner: Baked chicken, broccoli and corn on the cob.

Tracy suggested that I take a look at the food labels on the foods I was eating for breakfast. I was appalled to find that the granola bar had 20 grams of sugar and the nutrition shake had about the same amount. I was getting about 40 grams of sugar in one sitting and that's a lot of sugar. I learned that sugar, (glucose), turns to fat if it is not used. She also suggested that I add some snacks to my meal plan and that I watch my portion sizes.

Portion control is by far the biggest issue that Americans face with regard to weight loss. I am not a sponsor of eliminating entire food groups from your meal selections. I do believe that the majority of the foods we eat should be the seed-bearing plants (vegetables, fruits, grains and beans) because those are the first foods. The other portion can be devoted to lean cuts of meat and occasional treats. When you consume most meals, half of your plate should be vegetables and the other half should be meats and starches. Too often the biggest portion of our dinner plates is the meat or the carbohydrate. Your portions should be the size of your fist and the only foods you can add a little more too is the veggies.

Some have adopted the phrase, "all things in moderation," in terms of portion control and even eating unhealthy foods. That phrase is subjective to say the least. For example: to someone who eats fast food at every meal, a more moderate attempt would be to eat fast food once every day, which is still unhealthy. We are told in God's word that (1 Corinthians 10:23) all things are permissible, meaning you can eat whatever you want, but not all things are beneficial. If the purpose is to nourish your body, not to fulfill pleasurable desires or fill empty voids through food, then eating the foods that are best for you should not be an issue.

I began taking more precise notes about the portions in my food diary. This helped me to see that I was using more condiments than I needed to and that I was eating more than the serving size of some foods, therefore getting more calories than I thought. For example: One serving of Old Fashioned Oatmeal is one-half of a cup which is 150 calories, but I was eating over two cups in a serving. That means I was getting twice the calories. Here is what my food diary looked like when I started tracking portion size:

Day 1 Week 4:

- Breakfast – ½ cup of oatmeal with agave nectar and cinnamon with 1 cup orange juice
- Snack – Fat free yogurt cup with a glass of water
- Lunch – ½ Turkey sandwich on whole wheat bread with fat free cheese, lettuce and tomatoes with bottle of water
- Snack - ½ Turkey sandwich on whole wheat bread with fat free cheese, lettuce and tomatoes with bottle of water
- Dinner – Fist size portions of salmon, broccoli and brown rice with a glass of water and 1 cup of V8 V-Fusion® fruit juice

I received additional education on nutrition by watching Dr. Oz when he was a guest on *The Oprah Winfrey Show*. I learned some pivotal things that have helped me to make better choices at the grocery store. I would take notes because I was so serious about making improved choices and I would even share the things I learned with family and friends. I learned what my poop should look like and though that may sound nasty to you, what's even nastier is if you are not pooping at all. Before, I would only poop maybe once a week if that, today I am proud to say that I poop at least once every day.

For the moms and dads out there, you remember having a newborn baby and the doctor made you monitor the poop. Poop can tell you a lot about your body and whether you are getting the nutrients you need. It should not be uncomfortable and you should not have to strain. It should not be watery or hard but fluffy, and long.

Here are some things I learned about nutrition:

- **Eliminate high fructose corn syrup**

    This was very challenging. As I read the nutrition labels on the foods I had on my list, I noticed everything had high fructose corn syrup in it. The cereal I ate, the salad dressing, the peanut butter and even the ketchup. I had to find alternative options and that wasn't always easy. My quests sometimes lead me to buying organic options.

You might ask, "What's the big deal? What is high fructose corn syrup?" High fructose corn syrup is a scientifically created form of sugar, but studies have found that our bodies don't react to this sugar the same way it reacts to other sugars. "In the 40 years since the introduction of high-fructose corn syrup as a cost-effective sweetener in the American diet, rates of obesity in the U.S. have skyrocketed, according to the Centers for Disease Control and Prevention." [7]

High fructose corn syrup has been shown to cause increased weight gain. The problem is there are enough factors contributing to our obesity and weight gain. We want to eliminate as many culprits as possible.

- **Don't drink calories**.

    I did not prefer to drink water. I never understood the importance of drinking it. But I didn't prefer soda either. I loved juice. Grape juice was one of my favorites. I also loved strawberry flavored Kool-Aid®, a drink mix sold in packets, with at least three cups of sugar added to the pitcher.

    My mom is a coffee drinker and I have many friends that love the roasted beverage as well. A cup a day is okay but be mindful of what you add to it. Adding cream and sugar can turn a

---

[7] Hillary Parker, "A Sweet Problem: Princeton Researchers find that High-fructose Corn Syrup Prompts Considerably More Weight Gain." Princeton University, Mar 22, 2010. www.Princeton.edu.

smooth drink into a whole meal of 600 calories. The same is true with alcohol. Some wines, in particular red wine, have proven to have heart benefits but don't take it too far. These lively spirits can also load on the pounds. Having over three drinks can send you over the 2000 calorie a day mark. So just be mindful when drinking coffee and alcohol and make water the first choice.

This is one of the ways that we Americans can consume over 3000 calories in one day. When you drink a tall glass of juice or punch or have a bottle of soda, you are consuming a minimum of 200 calories. Now that's just once a day. Imagine how many calories you consume if you have three (600 calories) or four (800 calories). Most of us should be eating between 1800 to 2000 calories per day for women and 2300 to 2500 calories per day for men, depending on your level of activity. When you consume 800 calories alone in beverages, it leaves little room for you to get the nutrients you need from food.

- **Drink plenty of water each day.**

  Water has many functions in your body; all of them keep you living and thriving. Water helps regulate your body temperature and allows nutrients to travel through your body. Water also transports oxygen to your cells and removes waste. The blood in your body that's keeping you alive is made mostly of water.

  You lose water every day through urine, bowel movements, perspiration and your breath. The water that's lost is only replenished by consuming foods that contain water and by drinking water itself.

- **Always read food labels**

  Now this one takes some patience at the grocery store but it is gravely important. By reading labels I discovered that the foods that I thought were healthy were not healthy at all. I was being fooled by descriptions such as, "low-fat," "multi-grain," and "sugar free." None of these descriptions mean that these foods are healthy. Often times when they remove fat or sugar, they add something else that's just as bad.

It's also important to pay attention to the serving size. Let's say you grab an item that says only 100 calories per serving and 5 grams of fat. Sounds good, right? It only sounds good until you look at the fact that one serving is only 6 chips. So if you eat 12 chips you get 200 calories and 10 grams of fat. Always pay attention to the serving size.

The final reason you want to read nutrition labels is to know what you are eating. There's more to eating healthy than just paying attention to calories, fat and sugar. You also want to make sure you are eating natural foods; the foods God created for us. This is extremely difficult when it comes to packaged foods because they are man made.

It's always better to buy fresh foods, but when you want to buy snacks and cereals look for products whose ingredients include words that you can pronounce. If there are over 12 ingredients in one product I think you'd be safer to just leave it on the shelf.

- **Avoid trans-fat.**

    Trans-fats are not good for you. They raise your bad (LDL) cholesterol levels and lower your good (HDL) cholesterol levels. According to the American Heart Association, eating trans-fats increases your risk of developing heart disease and stroke. It's also associated with a higher risk of developing type 2 diabetes. [8]

[8] "Trans-fat," American Heart Association, www.Heart.org.

You may find that most labels and restaurants tout that they have 0 grams of trans-fats in their food or product. Just because a food package says no trans-fat does not mean it has zero grams of trans-fat, if it has partially hydrogenated oils in it those are trans-fats but because the amount is so low they are allowed to make this claim.

- **Replace the breads, rice and pastas with whole grains and brown rice.**

  One reason I immediately made the switch was to add fiber into my meals. Fiber helps us stay regular and helps support a healthy colon. It also lowers your risk of heart disease and diabetes. Whole grains provide an excellent source of fiber.

  White rice, white pastas and white breads are stripped of all the beneficial parts of the grain and then they attempt to add it back through enrichment. This is why you'll see, "enriched flour," on some food labels. When the nutrients are added back they are there but not nearly as beneficial to your body as if they were in their original form. By eating them, you are basically eating a depleted form of nutrients.

- **Use fat free or low-fat dairy products.**

  Since I started on my journey to healthy living, I have become lactose intolerant so at this point I don't consume dairy at all. If you are so blessed to be able to consume dairy, choose the fat free ones.

  Dairy has so many nutrients like vitamin D and calcium that so many of us don't get enough of. Unfortunately, dairy is also full of fat. Fats are not all bad. There are fats that are heart healthy and have omega 3 fatty acids in them like avocado, flax and extra virgin olive oil.

Eating too much fat, specifically the wrong kinds of fats, can increase our risk for high cholesterol, which can lead to heart disease and obesity. Choosing fat free or low-fat dairy is one sure way to limit your intake of high fat foods.

- **Avoid artificial sweeteners.**

As I write this, I picture my grandma squeezing lemon juice into her ice water and a pink packet of sugar substitute. Artificial sweeteners are hidden in many foods with names like aspartame and saccharin. The fact is researchers have not been able to prove that these chemically engineered sugars have any adverse affects and many are advocates of them because they are zero calorie foods. But just because something has not been proven does not mean that it is safe.

Critics believe, based on a study done in the 1970's with lab rats and saccharin, that these artificial sweeteners may be linked to cancer. [9]

Use agave nectar or honey as a sweetener instead of artificial sweeteners. These are things from the earth that God made for us. Anything made in a lab or made through some chemical process is not the best choice.

Overall, you want to limit your sugar intake all together even when you choose the natural sugars. Eating too much added sugar increases your chances for diabetes and heart disease.

There are naturally occurring sugars in fruits, whole grains, veggies and low fat dairy products. These foods contain essential nutrients that we need. Added sugars are empty nutrients, meaning that they have no nutritional benefit.

---

[9] Elena Conis, "Saccharin's Mostly Sweet Following," *Los Angeles Times*. Dec 27, 2010. www.LaTimes.com.

Look for these names when searching for sugar on a nutrition label:

- Dextrose
- Brown sugar
- Corn sweetener
- Corn syrup
- Fructose
- Molasses
- Corn sugar
- Maltose
- Sucrose
- Sucralose
- Honey
- Malt syrup
- High-fructose corn syrup
- Glucose
- Lactose
- Raw sugar
- Brown rice syrup
- Syrup

- **Eat at least five small meals a day.**

     When I say five meals I don't mean five large plates of food. The idea is to graze and eat smaller meals throughout the day so that you never become overly hungry. When we let our bodies get to a place where we are extremely hungry, we usually eat so fast that we overeat.

     Eating smaller meals throughout the day also helps to speed up your metabolism. Eating this way helps to stabilize blood sugar levels and this is important because large rises in blood sugar levels can promote the production of insulin which can lead to the storage of fat.

• **Watch the salt.**

Because we eat so much packaged and processed foods, our sodium intakes are off the charts. For the fun of it, my husband looked at the nutritional information for a number of 'healthy restaurants.' We were surprised to see that the most of the sandwiches and foods that we once loved had as much as 3500 mg of sodium. That is outrageous!

Eating too much salt can cause your body to retain water, which can prevent weight loss, but it can also cause high blood pressure which can lead to heart disease. The *2010 Dietary Guidelines for Americans* recommends limiting sodium to less than 2,300 mg a day—1,500 mg if you're over age 51, if you are black, or if you have high blood pressure, diabetes or chronic kidney disease. [10]

While we need sodium, having it in excess is never a good thing. Limit your salt intake by cooking at home, using fresh foods as much as possible, cooking with natural herbs and spices instead of salt and using low sodium products.

• **Drive by the drive-thru.**

We've all grown up on burger and French fry serving fast food restaurants and for whatever reason many of us can't be pulled away from there. Fast food is designed to be fast. In most cases, when things are done faster, they are not always

---

[10] "Sodium: How to Tame your Salt Habit Now." *Mayo Clinic*, www.mayoclinic.com.

done properly. Most of the items on the menu of fast food joints are high in unhealthy fat, sugar and sodium. All three being things that our bodies should never have in excess.

While many fast food restaurants offer, "healthier," options, these choices are still high in sodium and many contain added preservatives to make up for the ingredients they took out to make the food lower in fat.

Don't be fooled by restaurants that claim to be healthier or even organic. My husband and I were fans of two or three fast food chains that made these claims. When we went on their websites to look at their nutrition facts and ingredients, there was nothing healthy about them. The menu items were full of salt and sugar—as much as 50g of sugar in one item. When we want fast food we opt for Subway® sandwich shop or Chick-fil-A® fast food chicken restaurant. Chick-fil-A® has a very healthy children's menu that features grilled chicken nuggets and fruit salads. They also offer fresh romaine lettuce on their grilled chicken sandwich and salad as a side.

Having a sit down meal at a restaurant is not always the better choice either. Many of their ingredients are prepackaged and frozen and then cooked in oil and butter. They also contain large amounts of sodium and fat. What's your best bet? Eat at home. When you prepare your own food you ensure that you and your family are getting the very best.

- **Grill or bake meats as opposed to frying.**
  Being born and raised in the South, I have had my share of fried chicken and fried pork chops. While these foods are tantalizingly tasty, they also pose health risks if eaten habitually.

The problem with fried foods is that they contain those pesky trans-fats that we talked about earlier. They also contain saturated fats. These are not the good fats that you need and can again lead to high cholesterol and heart disease.

Try baking your meats instead. If you just have to have fried foods, try oven frying or air baking.

- **Eat carbs.**

This may sound unorthodox to some who have been successful losing weight by cutting carbs (carbohydrates) or removing them entirely from your diet. But carbohydrates are important for our bodies. They provide our bodies with energy.

When we say carbs we need to make some distinctions. Some prefer simplifying them into the categories of simple and complex. Complex carbs include whole grains, brown rice and beans for example. Fruit, veggies and dairy products are all simple carbs, but they are also packed with nutrients. On the other hand, refined sugars are simple carbs as well and they can be found in candy, cakes and other snacks with added sugar.

It was once thought that the simpler a carbohydrate is, the faster the body absorbs it. The more complex it is, the longer it takes to digest. The faster the process of digestion; the higher spike in blood sugar levels. However, some foods that are considered complex like starches, also raise blood sugar levels. You always want to keep your blood sugar level steady because this prevents us from craving foods and suffering from feelings of hunger. High blood sugar levels increase ones chances for diabetes, heart disease and atherosclerosis.

Another way to look at carbs is according to their Glycemic Index (GI), which classifies foods according to how quickly they raise blood sugar levels. There are low, medium and high glycemic index foods. We want to eat mostly low glycemic index foods like whole oats, apples and chickpeas (fruits, veggies, legumes and whole grains that are minimally processed), whereas those with a high glycemic index include corn chips, jelly beans and breakfast cereals.

It can all be a tad bit confusing I'm sure. But remember at the end of the day you want to eat whole grains, lean meats, veggies, fruits, beans, and nuts. As my grandma used to say, "Eat lots of green leafy veggies." Those have so many benefits. And while the "typical" fruits are good, (apples, oranges and bananas), other fruits are just as good like strawberries and blueberries that offer antioxidants which help fight disease and infection. Fruits are higher in sugar, some more than others, so just be mindful. You should be eating more veggies than fruits.

They key is to find balance in the foods that you eat. Never remove an entire food group from your food selection. Eat more (lots) of the first foods and less of the foods man created because more and more what we are discovering is that the best foods for our bodies are the foods that naturally occur on earth.

❖ Bonus Tip ❖

Eat slowly and be aware of the food you are eating. Sometimes it takes a bit longer for your brain to let your stomach know it is full. If you eat slower and chew longer, your tummy will get the memo before you've over eaten.

* * * * * *

Another step I took toward becoming educated in nutrition and exercise was reading fitness magazines. Now this was hard for me initially and it eventually led to me starting my own magazine. The fitness magazines often feature half-naked women on their covers. Flipping through the magazines was discouraging because all the women and men in the magazine were extremely fit. Why weren't there people that were struggling with weight? Why weren't there any people who were average-sized? I left the magazine aisle feeling inadequate, but I did learn some exercises I could do at home and some cool recipes that I could integrate into my meal plan. The most important thing I learned from reading those magazines is that protein fuels muscles and too often we don't get enough protein each day.

About 10% of the foods that you eat should be proteins so if you eat 2,000 calories per day, you should consume 200 calories of protein. There are 4 calories in a gram of protein so that would be about 50 grams. I noticed that when I ate more protein, I kept the weight off and my muscles continued to tone. To get the grams that I need each day, I usually make a smoothie for lunch with protein powder. I also try to incorporate protein into each meal and snack.

I pondered, "With God being the God that He is, He had to give us some directions on food." In my Bible Study and time with the Lord one morning I came across this scripture in the book of Genesis chapter one and verse twenty-nine, "Then God said, "I give you every seed-bearing plant on the face of the whole earth and every tree that has fruit with seed in it. They will be yours for food." Here we see that when we were created, God intended for us to eat only vegetables, beans, grains and fruit; seed-bearing plants. When I saw this I then began to understand why our bodies require these foods the most. We see this again in Genesis 1:30, which says, "And to all the beasts of the earth and all the birds of the air and all the creatures that move on the ground—everything that has the breath of life in it—I give every green plant for food." Not only did God give us these foods to eat, but He gave it to all the other creatures that He created. These were the first foods.

Having this revelation helped me to mend my mind about my desire for these foods because I believe that if these are the original foods that God gave us as food to eat, there must be a reason. If they were good for us then, they are good for us now. It wasn't until after the flood that God gave us animals to eat (Genesis 9:3) and then He later gave us instructions on which meats we should and shouldn't eat in Leviticus 11.

Once I learned what foods to eat, I also had to become skilled at how to season them. I use Mrs. Dash® seasonings, herbs for meats, and agave nectar or unsweetened apple sauce for baking or sweetening. My taste buds began to become accustomed to these new foods. Trust me yours will too. My husband used to love salty foods. Did I mention that he is from New Orleans? But now, when he tastes something overly salty, he notices it immediately. It's because your taste buds adjust to the foods you eat on a consistent basis. You will no longer want the same foods you used to eat and in most cases your body won't take them. What do I mean? After starting to eat healthier, I hadn't had a soda in a while and decided that I wanted a taste. I took a sip and I thought my mouth was on fire. My throat felt like it was burning and I haven't had a soda since. Another example is when my husband and I, after not having eaten fried meat for a while, decided to go have some hot wings. Let's just say the toilet was a, "shoulder," that we both leaned on that night.

The reality is the healthier foods won't taste just like the other versions that you are used to. Most people think that turkey bacon is not nearly as flavorful as pork bacon. I think you'd do yourself an injustice by expecting the alternatives to taste like the other foods you are used to. No, fat free cheese is not going to taste like whole milk cheese and a brownie made with applesauce instead of sugar won't taste like a regular brownie. But remember that you control your body, it does not control you. You tell your body, "You will like these foods because they are better for you." It's all in perspective. Just because something tastes different does not mean it's nasty. Renew your taste buds by introducing them to healthier foods and renew your mind by welcoming those new tastes!

* * * *

A Renewed Outlook on Exercise

I was just as ignorant in the area of exercise as I was when it came to food. I did not know a thing. All I knew was to get on a machine whether it was a treadmill or a bike. I just knew that I needed to be sweating and panting for air. I thought that lifting weights was only for people who wanted to be big and bulky, and because I did not want to look like that I stayed away from weights. Again, I had to change my thinking and repair my mind in this area because what I eventually learned was that strength training was just as important as cardiovascular training. Why? Because muscle actually burns fat, so as you build muscle by strength training, you burn fat and your muscles become more toned.

Most people who hit the gym and have never hired a trainer or been properly educated on exercise, are "either or people." They either prefer cardio or they favor strength training. Both are equally important. In essence, cardio or aerobic training is strength training because you are working one of the most important muscles in your body, your heart.

There are different ways to strength train. You can use free weights (dumbbells), machines or resistance bands. I prefer machines for leg work and free weights for arm work. I noticed that as I did more strength training not only did I see results, but I saw definition in my arms, legs and butt. Don't think that you have to go to the gym either, with some resistance bands or dumbbells; you can get a great work out right in your living room.

If you decide to join a gym, please pay careful attention to the introductory tour they give you when you first join. They should tell you about all the machines and which machines work which body parts. I recommend that you take advantage of the free personal training session as well because they will teach you how to do each exercise properly. While exercising is a great thing, it's imperative that you are doing the exercises properly to prevent injuries, especially weight bearing exercises. One exercise that I always did wrong was the squat. Doing this exercise wrong can damage your knees. You would be surprised at the thousands of injuries that occur at gyms on a daily basis due to improper form.

One important thing I learned was to warm up before exercising and stretch after exercising. I see this mistake every day at the gym. People want to jump right into exercising. Exercising cold muscles can increase your chance of injury. A proper warm up prepares your body for the activity and gradually raises body temperature and increases blood flow to the muscles. A warm up can simply be a five minute brisk walk or some jumping jacks. The point is to prepare the body for the activity.

Stretching after exercise is also important and often overlooked. Stretching can help prevent injury, increase flexibility, and even improve performance. But stretches can also be dangerous if not done properly. I suggest seeking a professional to teach you the basics of stretching.

Here are some tips:

- Never bounce.
- It should not be painful.
- Stretch the muscles you've used.

* * * *

Motivation

After reading all of that you may still be thinking, "I want my pork bacon and I want my Coke and I really don't feel like exercising." The bottom line is there is no book, program or pill that is going to change you. You have to decide that you want the change and that you are ready to make the change. Until then, you are wasting your time and money. Find something to motivate you. My motivation came when my mom who was in her early forties at the time, was near stroke level because of her high cholesterol. I also learned that my dad had high blood pressure and although the doctors weren't sure, they believed he had had a stroke because his mouth was twisted. That was enough to motivate me. I refused to depend on medications for the rest of my life to control something that I could very well control myself. That's when I decided to hire a personal trainer and at least try to lose weight.

If that doesn't motivate you, look into the eyes of your children and/or the people that love you. Visualize what life would be like for them without you. They love you and they need you. Heart disease is often a silent killer, but unfortunately it's the number one cause of death in America. I'm sorry to say this but it could be you, and you don't want to leave your family that way. Live for them.

Above everything do it for you! Aren't you worth it? Don't you deserve to be healthy and whole? If you answered no let me tell you, you are worth it. You are a child of God and God loves you. He has a purpose and a plan for you. He sent His son Jesus just for you. Jesus died so that we might live abundantly (John 10:10). Being overweight and unhealthy is not the abundant life and it is therefore not what Jesus died for. Honor his sacrifice and live the abundant life by taking care of yourself!

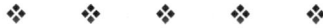

❖   ❖   ❖   ❖   ❖

TINY TIP:
If you're having a hard time sticking to a workout regimen, perhaps you haven't found your niche. Try dancing, kettle bell workouts, or even water aerobics! Keep it spicy and you'll keep at it!

Prayer:

Father, I come to you asking that you would help me to renew my mind. Help me to use your Word to reshape the way I think about eating and exercise. Let your Word change the way I feel about the way I treat this temple (my body). I am ready for change. I am ready to make a difference in my health and therefore in my life. Deliver me from any strongholds that might be stopping me from living a healthy lifestyle and surround me with people that will encourage and motivate me.

Thank you for a new outlook and a new attitude. I will eat the foods that are most beneficial to my body and I will become physically active for you said it was of value.

I praise you in advance for helping me to lose weight, but more importantly I thank you for showing me that if I trust and depend on you with pure motives, I can accomplish anything.

In Jesus' Name,
Amen

ℛ ℭ

RENEWED

My mind is renewed

like the sun

As it makes its first peak upon

A cloud.

My eyes have been reopened

Like a baby's first look

Outside the womb.

Everything looks new,

smells new,

tastes new,

Happier thoughts overcome me,

as I look ahead.

I'm a new person,

the old one is dead.

ℛ ℭ

ഇരു

CHAPTER 7
ഇരു

Making Fitness a Lifestyle

Everything is permissible —
but not everything is beneficial.
Everything is permissible — but
not everything is constructive.

1 Corinthians 10:23

ॐ ଓ

It didn't take long before I understood why Tracy was disinclined to introduce me to calorie counting. I took it and ran with it. I was determined to lose weight, no matter the cost. I started counting each and every calorie that I ate and I wrote it in my food diary. By then I was also working out twice a day. When I had surpassed my goal of getting down to 127 lbs., that goal was no longer good enough. I felt like I needed to lose more if I really wanted to look like, "the picture."

It was my great idea to cut out a picture of what I wanted to look like and look at it along with my scripture reading and meditation each morning. The picture I chose happened to be a picture of the actress, Halle Berry. Even when I was at a healthy weight, I still did not look like "the picture." Wanting to look like that was an unrealistic goal and it just proves that my mind still needed a bit more renewing. But would I ever look like that picture?

Here is the problem when we compare ourselves to others. Our bodies are unique and different. Some women have more defined curves, while others don't. Some men have more defined muscles naturally, while others don't. But that does not make one body type better than the other. It just means they are different. You have to learn to appreciate the body that you were given.

It's just like when I share my weight loss testimony with others. Some think that just because my "number" was smaller than their number; somehow my testimony is less potent. At my biggest I was 160 lbs. and no, that is not huge, but relatively speaking for my five foot one frame, it was a lot of weight for me to carry. My ankles ached, I had back aches and as I mentioned before, I was having heart palpitations. I could not make it up a flight of stairs without taking a break and I was only eighteen years old. The number is not the issue. The issue is that we all need to be healthier. When you view weight loss this way, you have an unhealthy attitude about health because the goal is not to get down to a certain size rather it is to be healthy.

I wanted to look like, "the picture," so I cut my calories down to 1600 per day. Now for some who are moderately active this might be a good amount of energy (calories = energy) for you, but at the time I was working out rigorously twice a day. My husband, who by now was a personal trainer, trained me on the days when Tracy didn't. He helped me to get past my plateau and taught me exercises that I could do at home. He also taught me how to run, something that I had always despised.

Get Support

One of the biggest blessings that I had during this journey of losing weight was the support of my husband. He was on board and encouraged me. For others that I've met at gyms, they look to their personal trainers for support and extra pushing. No matter where you find it, you need support. You need someone there to keep you motivated and hold you accountable on the days when you just don't feel like exercising. This is why programs like Weight Watchers® (if you take advantage of the meetings) are so great because they allow you to get around other people and form a support system. I would say that for me this and God's word were the main reasons why I was able to lose weight and maintain the weight loss.

"Well, Arian I don't have a husband to support me and I can't afford a trainer or a fancy weight loss program. What do I do?" You might ask. Seek help. My grandmother used to tell me, "Closed mouths don't get fed." This means that people who just sit there waiting for something to happen never see it happen. When you want something you have to be willing to seek out the resources you need. There are tons of churches in our country that now have fitness programs and classes, and often times you don't have to be a member. There are also meet up groups (meetup.com) that meet and walk every day and if there is not one in your area, maybe you can start one. In the summer time, there are even free boot camps at local parks on Saturday mornings. In Joshua 1:8 we are told that we should make our way prosperous, first by meditating on the word of God and then by acting out on the faith that we obtain by meditating on that word. We are told that faith without works is dead (James 2:17). If you want to be successful in the area of health and fitness, make your way prosperous by acting out on your motivational scripture through faith and getting yourself hooked up with people who will support you and see you through to your goal.

When my support system was no longer around (my husband was deployed in the military), my vision became distorted. The mission to lose weight overpowered my desire to be healthy and to honor God with my body. I remember getting down to 113 lbs. and that may sound wonderful to you, but allow me to let you take a peek at what I was doing to get to that weight. Here's my diet. Notice when I refer to nourishment throughout this book I use meal plan or meal options, instead of diet, but this was a diet. Why? Because I could have very well die-d from my die-t. I was eating 1200 calories per day and exercising twice a day.

Food Diary Entry:

- Breakfast – One waffle with peanut butter and banana
- Snack – 12 almonds

- Lunch – Fruit smoothie made with ½ cup soy milk, 3 cup strawberries and blue berries and a serving of soy protein with ice
- Snack – One kiwi
- Dinner – One lean, frozen dinner and a spinach smoothie

I would wake up and work out first thing in the morning before work and then I would take a vigorous walk during my lunch hour. I was so frail. Because I had a picture of myself at my heaviest weight of 160 lbs., I would look at the picture and think, "I'm never going back." Any weight gain would send me to tears because I was so afraid of going back to my old weight. Fear was one of the things that drove me, and as Christians we are to be driven by love, not fear.

If I ate too much, I would work out even harder and I hopped on the scale every morning and every night. I remember crying one afternoon to my husband when the scale showed that I had gained a pound. I had equated my self-worth to the numbers that showed up on the scale. That day I didn't measure up.

If I ate something that was unhealthy like ice cream or cake, I would feel guilty. The guilt would cause me to eat even less. It also affected my walk with God. I felt condemned. Condemnation only comes to make us feel inferior and undeserving. Simply put, it's one of the enemy's avenues of separating us away from the Father and away from fellow believers. When we go before God, we must go boldly and with confidence. 1 John 5:14 says, "This is the confidence we have in approaching God: that if we ask anything according to His will, he hears us." When we allow guilt to creep in, we destroy our confidence. Having a treat every now and then should not bring on guilt. If you fall into gluttony, simply repent, leave it alone and take on a new thought. Don't stay there.

I became addicted to losing weight. This is what happens when we don't deal with the root of addictions, they simply transfer to other areas of our lives. I hadn't dealt with the reason why I was overweight, so when I began losing weight, the obsessive behavior that was a result of the pains and hurts from my past shifted to my weight loss. Neither being overweight or obsessed with losing weight is a healthy way of life, for being healthy is about having balance, not operating in extremes. Ecclesiastes 7:16-19 says, "Do not be overrighteous, neither be overwise—why destroy yourself? Do not be overwicked, and do not be a fool—why die before your time? It is good to grasp the one and not let go of the other. The man who fears God will avoid all extremes." In this scripture Solomon helps us understand that we should avoid extremes and instead seek balance in our lives.

I had to learn that fitness was not about losing weight. It's not even about maintaining a certain weight. Fitness is a lifestyle. It's the way you live every day. We cannot be so caught up in our outer appearance that we forsake our spiritual health. 3 John 1:2 KJV says, "Beloved, I wish above all things that thou mayest prosper and be in health, even as thy soul prospereth." As your soul prospers so will your body and the other areas of your life. But your soul is not prospering if you are in bondage to eating disorders, not eating enough to sustain you or eating more than what your body needs for nourishment. Remember, we are losing weight because we want to be healthy so we can live long and carry out God's will for our lives, not to look a certain way.

Deal with the issue. We talked about this before but I want to reiterate how important it is to deal with your issues related to food. Don't let overcoming one thing lead you to an addiction to something else. You have a blood bought right to deliverance. Know that you do not have to suffer with any addictions or bondage because of the price that Jesus paid. Nothing can hold you captive. You have been set free! Accept your deliverance and receive it by the blood of Jesus.

Recite this declaration:

> I declare by and through the blood of Jesus that I am delivered from an addiction to food, to drugs, to weight loss and to any other external things. I am free to live in abundant health; whole and disease free. I am healed from my past and I leave those things behind, pressing forward for what God has in store for me. I love myself and I believe that I am good enough. Today, I declare that living healthy is my new lifestyle. I am fit and ready for the Maker's use.

> **Scripture Reference**: "Don't grieve God. Don't break his heart. His Holy Spirit, moving and breathing in you, is the most intimate part of your life, making you FIT for himself." (Ephesians 4:30 MSG)

My vision became distorted not only because my husband was away at sea, but more importantly, because I stopped renewing my mind. I ditched meditating on my scriptures and seeking God for help. I stopped praying and worshiping during my exercise routines and workouts. After getting so far in my weight loss, I took on the, "I've arrived," attitude. We never arrive. We are always reliant upon God for strength. Our minds are not renewed, but they are renewing each day. Once I realized this I got back on board, meditating and confessing, specifically in the area of my health.

* * * *

Finding Balance

I remember when I would have those moments of condemnation I would go to the altar and have ministers pray for me. I would have them pray for my deliverance. What I did not understand at that time was that I had already been delivered. I needed to walk in that deliverance. The same way you have to work out your own salvation (Philippians 2:12), you also have to work out your deliverance. You work out your deliverance by setting up boundaries that will assist you in making this a lifestyle.

The way a porn addict sets up blockers on his computer, you should also arrange your life so that temptation is not readily available. The steps that I took were:

- Never bringing food into the house that I would overindulge in (ice cream and chocolate).
- Talking to other people about health and fitness (Trust me; other people will hold you accountable. They see you slipping and they will ask, "I thought you were a health freak?"
- Designating one day a week as a treat day.

The biggest help was not bringing tempting foods in the house. When I would have bad days and I just wanted to shove a whole gallon of ice cream down my throat, I was left eating an apple.

I had to learn to make fitness a part of my life and understand that fitness is not my life. I went from exercising six days a week, twice a day, to exercising five days a week, once a day. I tried to vary my exercises so I would not become bored with them. Getting uninterested is the reason some people just stop exercising altogether. Please know that going to the gym is not the only way that you can stay active. There are tons of non-traditional methods of exercising: swimming, dancing and karate are all activities that you can do to get moving. Find something that you enjoy doing and stick to that and when it gets boring try something else. One exercise craze that is taking America by storm is Zumba® and I recommend it for anyone that is just getting into fitness. It's fun and it works off the pounds.

I learned not to focus on being a certain weight, but to endeavor to be healthy. I went from counting calories to not counting at all. I went from being condemned after eating a slice of cake to having a treat once a week and actually looking forward to it. I learned not to be so uptight about every little thing. I remember looking back and laughing because my husband and I went to a cookout at my job and I brought my own ketchup and my own bread just in case they didn't have wheat bread and their ketchup had high fructose corn syrup in it. I had it all packaged up and pulled it out proudly as we sat at a picnic table with unbelieving onlookers. That was laughable. Having these things sometimes is okay. Besides, at least they had veggie and turkey burgers at the cookout. I had to relax and just enjoy life. I got tired of measuring every little thing. When I lived away from my hometown, I remember visiting my mom and measuring one cup of cereal. I then measured my milk and the amount of fruit that I put in the cereal. Being so anal about fitness made it unrealistic to maintain. If it's going to be a way of life it has to be manageable.

At the present, I eat about 1800 calories per day and I know that, not because I count but, because I have a more conscious awareness of the foods that I put into my mouth. I feel good about myself and where I am in my health. I look in the mirror and I feel comfortable with my body. I either go for a run, hit the gym or do a workout DVD, which ever I choose I try to do some activity five days a week. I enjoy exercising and I look forward to it. It has become my stress reliever and we all need one of those. Even as I write this book, just yesterday a friend of mine who hasn't seen me in years said, "You've put on some weight." As inappropriate as her comment was, it didn't bother me. I didn't feel substandard or inadequate. Just a few years ago that comment would have sent me to the gym or had me crying to my husband about how fat I was.

A day in my meal plan today looks something like this:

- Breakfast – Kashi® Go Lean® whole grain cereal with Almond Milk
- Snack – One serving almonds
- Lunch – Turkey sandwich on whole grain bread with lettuce and tomatoes and Sun Chips® multi-grain chips
- Snack – An apple with peanut butter
- Dinner – Fist size servings of salmon, sweet potato and spinach
- Snack – protein bar

Today I am at peace and content. That does not mean that I have arrived. Again, we never arrive and we never reach perfection. Jesus was the only perfect one. Some people struggle with weight issues and eating problems for the rest of their lives. I still desire sweets when I'm sad or alone, but the difference is that I know why I am craving those things and I make a conscious effort to redirect my mind. Since there aren't any tempting foods in my house, I usually have to just suck it up and get over it. I've also gotten back to my prayers for help during exercise and meditating on scriptures throughout the day. Fitness is a journey; you will have different seasons in your life. The key is continuously making health a priority and making God your source of strength.

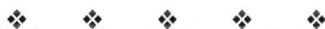

❖   ❖   ❖   ❖   ❖

TINY TIP:
Don't identify yourself with being overweight. Be unique! 70% of Americans are obese or overweight. Don't fit in, get fit!

Prayer:

Lord I am ready for this journey of living a healthy lifestyle. I am willing to make whatever changes I need to make to honor your temple in my eating and exercise. I will make fitness a part of my everyday life. Help me Lord. I recognize that I need you. Be my strength, Lord.

Lead and guide me towards an activity that I will enjoy. Help me to stay active and not allow anything to distract me from honoring you with my body. Help me to set up boundaries in my life so that I will honor you in my eating.

I declare victory today over my health and wellness and I move forward boldly and in confidence.

In Jesus' Name,
Amen

A LIFESTYLE CHOICE

Every day I make the choice
To treat my body right,
No longer will I abuse it
For its precious in His sight.

I wake up every morning
With a desire to be well,
The things I eat and my activities,
Keep me feeling swell.

I'm no saint, I still mess up,
Perfection is never attained
But I keep going and I keep at it,
Striving to maintain.

ഐ രൂ

CHAPTER 8

ഐ രൂ

Intimidated by Exercise

For God has not given us the spirit of fear; but of power, and of love, and of a sound mind.

2 Timothy 1:7 NKJV

∞ ∞

Walking into a gym for the first time reminded me of my first day of high school; everything and everyone seemed like giants. I was intimidated by all of the equipment and the machines that rattled and beeped. I was unsettled by the huge, bulky men gasping and moaning as they pressed weights to their chest, and oh, how demoralized I was, by the women in their teeny, tiny workout clothes.

The music was reminiscent of a night club and the gym vaguely reminded me of my clubbing days, sweaty smells and people checking each other out. Every machine was in use and every class was full. "What have I gotten myself into?" I thought to myself. I'd be better off just walking around my neighborhood.

Once again I found myself in a situation where I felt alone and isolated. After spending a few minutes in the locker room, convincing myself that I was just as good as any of the people out on the gym floor, I eventually got enough guts to at least try to exercise. I found a corner treadmill and started walking. That's all I knew how to do.

Many of you have the very same feeling about going to the gym or even exercise altogether. You feel like it's for gym heads or for people who have had some special training. Going to the gym is only overwhelming the first time you go. Just like the first day of high school. By the next week, not only are you excited to go, but you have found your way around and met some friends to talk to.

When you sign up for a gym membership you should get a tour of the gym and a free session with a personal trainer. During that session, the trainer should do some fitness tests on you and help you determine what your fitness goals should be.

After I went through this test recently (we joined a new gym) the trainer told me, although I was physically fit, I needed to work on my balance and core strength. This is to be expected as I just had a baby the year before. He showed me some exercises that would help me to reach the goal of better balance. He also gave me a gym calendar and went through the classes the gym offered that might be good for me to take.

You should experience something similar at any gym. If you are already a member of a gym and have questions, utilize the staff and trainers that are standing around. Although they get paid by the hour, they are usually friendly people that don't mind answering a question or two about a machine.

I know economically, many of us can't afford to hire a personal trainer in addition to the monthly fee that we are already paying at the gym. I understand, but I do want to point out that there are some advantages to hiring a trainer. A trainer is your employee. Their job is to help you reach your physical best so the entire session of activity will be dedicated to you. Most importantly, a personal trainer can teach you the proper techniques for some exercises, how to warm up and how to stretch properly. Your body is a precious gift and there is a certain way you have to prepare it for activity and a way to bring it down from the workout.

You want to make sure that you get a good trainer. There are thousands of personal trainers out there, but not all of them are good nor do they all have your best interest at heart. Remember that you are paying them so you should be able to ask questions and request specific workouts. If a personal trainer does not do a fitness screening and test on you, how can they create a personalized plan for you? I recommend you observe a trainer in the act of training someone else so you can identify their personality and determine if it best suits you. Some trainers are more harsh than others; some are calm motivators while others like to bring the pain and have no mercy for weakness.

A good trainer should also be able to tell you which exercises work which muscles and which exercises are best for your specific goals. Their goal should be to get you started on a regular exercise plan and teach you variety so that eventually you can do it on your own. Most importantly, they should be certified and have insurance.

If you cannot afford a trainer and it's simply out of the question, take some of the classes. Gyms have everything from boot camps to spin classes. They also have yoga, water aerobics and kickboxing and these classes are totally free for members.

Here are some popular gym classes:

- **Spin Class** – an hour class done on stationary bikes. This is a high intensity class and burns hundreds of calories.
- **Boot Camp** – an hour class of cardio drills, strength training and body weight exercises.
- **Water Aerobics** – an hour of aerobic activity done in the shallow area of the pool. This class works the entire body at one time and it is perfect for any age.
- **Yoga** – an hour class that helps improve flexibility and balance. It also helps with posture.
- **Kickboxing** – an hour class that utilizes the punches of boxing and the kicks of karate. It is a combination of aerobics, martial arts and boxing. This is a high intensity class.
- **Zumba®** – a Latin inspired dance class that incorporates movement of all major body parts.
- **Cross Fit** – a high intensity workout designed to improve one's

ability to carry out physically challenging tasks. It will improve stamina and endurance.

- **Pilates** – an hour class that develops core strength and flexibility. It also focuses a lot on breathing.

One of the classes that I took when I first joined a gym was the boot camp class. This is perfect for beginners in my opinion because you learn a variety of workouts. I admit that it's a bit higher in intensity, but instructors should provide alternative moves for people of all fitness levels.

So many of us who have never joined a gym only know about running or walking outside, or on a treadmill for exercise. There is so much more to it than that. Cardiovascular exercise, referred to as cardio, means that the main muscle you are working is your heart. Cardio exercises include running, jogging, walking briskly, etc.

However, it's a shame though that so many people, women especially, limit their physical activity to just cardio. Strength training is just as important for the body. It keeps your bones strong as they age. Strength training also helps to burn fat. It is not true that strength training will make you bulky. What is true is the more muscle mass you have the less fat you will have. This is why BMI measures your body mass index (how much of your body is fat).

It was in a boot camp class that I discovered my love for strength training. This is the key to making exercise a part of your lifestyle; finding something that you love, something that you could do every day.

Strength training means exactly what it sounds like; its training to increase strength. Strength training exercises can include the use of body weight (pushups), dumbbells or free weights (bench press) and resistance bands.

I prefer dumbbells because they allow more variety and movement for me, but resistance bands are awesome for beginners. They are also easy to transport so you can get in a few strength moves on your lunch break at work.

You probably do strength training exercises and don't even know it. As I mentioned before pushups are a type of strength developing exercise, as are squats and lunges. I implore you to add strength training into your physical activity.

Get Out of the Gym

Get out of the gym and create your own workout! My husband and I found going to the gym to sometimes be a chore so we bought some equipment of our own. We bought an elliptical machine and a Bowflex®. This way we could exercise right at home and not have to get up, get dressed and walk or drive to a gym. In the end, it's also a cost saver when you think of the money you'd spend being a member of a gym for a few years. We also bought some dumbbells and resistance bands.

When I needed a switch from the Bowlfex® home gym and elliptical machine, I would exercise with my workout DVD's. For me working out to the DVD's was like taking an aerobics class. I felt like I was there with the rest of the crew. The first one I used was the Power 90® workout program by Tony Horton. This was a good one to start out with because Tony Horton is pretty funny to me. Exercise should be fun. It's also more of a beginner style workout.

Going to the gym or using a home gym is not the only way to exercise. If you can't afford a gym membership or to create a home gym, there are other alternatives. I interviewed Dominique Dawes, an Olympic medalist, for the magazine and she said some things that resonated with me. As fit as she is, when I asked her about her workout regimen, she said that she didn't have one.

Imagine that! A woman whose entire career revolved around physical activity, did not have a weekly routine. What she said was that sometimes she goes to the gym, sometimes she just goes for a jog.

I've incorporated this attitude into my lifestyle. Sometimes I take a Zumba® class; sometimes I just put my son in his stroller and go for a walk. The idea of activity is to be active; not to kill ourselves at the gym every day. When we do that it becomes mundane and boring and we lose our motivation to exercise at all. Keeping it fresh helps us to keep moving. My husband does this. Every week he has a new routine otherwise, he doesn't have the desire to workout.

As a family, we like to find a nature trail and walk briskly. Inhaling fresh air is so relaxing. You can talk about your dreams and goals while you walk. You can talk about the love of God and how good He has been to you. You can praise Him while you walk; glorifying Him for all His marvelous works as you notice the trees and birds He created. Walking is an excellent aerobic activity.

Dancing is another great way to get your body moving and you won't even realize that you are exercising. Some local community centers even offer free dance classes or inexpensive ones. One that I've been interested in (but just haven't had the chance to try) is Salsa dancing. It seems young and sexy and we all like that!

Mix it up, keep it fresh and don't be intimidated. It's your body, now move it!

Learn Your Body

If you don't know what exercise works what body parts, you could be doing the wrong thing and working the wrong muscle groups. Knowing these muscles will also help you be able to read the exercise instructions on the machines at the gym.

Some of the major muscles that we focus on in exercise are biceps (front upper arm), triceps (back upper arm), quadriceps (front of thigh), calves (lower back leg), hamstrings (back of thigh), pectoralis major and minor (chest), gluteus maximus and minimus (butt), deltoids (shoulders), lattissmus dosi (back) and abdominals (stomach).

Become familiar with your body, learn about the muscle groups and all its wonderful parts!

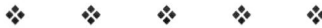

❖   ❖   ❖   ❖   ❖

TINY TIP:
Don't feel inferior when you go to the gym and see others lifting more weight or running faster than you. Do what works for you! Be authentic in your exercise!

Prayer:

Lord I thank you that I am no longer afraid to exercise. I'm not intimidated by the thought of going to the gym or the thought of getting active. I thank you that you will lead me to the right activity for me; that I will enjoy it and be able to make physical activity a part of my life.

I praise you for your faithfulness and seeing me to this point. Although I haven't been as active as I should, or take care of my body like I should, you have sustained me, for I am alive.

I thank you that I am able to exercise; that I have the mobility of my limbs and can move without the assistance of someone else. Help me to keep that in mind as I move on towards living healthier, pressing on towards the mark of the high calling.

In Jesus' Name,
Amen

IT WON'T MOVE

Tried on the jeans I once loved
The button flew across the room.
I have to get to the gym soon.

Joined a gym and never went
Too many people, too much equipment,
Money I should have never spent.

This big ole butt,
It won't leave,
This doggone gut,
It won't move,

Seeing a trainer tomorrow,
Gotta get in the groove.

ಋಾ ಲ

CHAPTER 9
ಋಾ ಲ

Food Panic

Do not be anxious about
anything, but in everything,
by prayer and petition, with
thanksgiving, present your
requests to God.

Philippians 4:6

ॐ ॲ

When I lost weight, I was on such a strict diet. I was so thin that it just didn't look good and my head looked too big. I remember when a certain celebrity attorney lost weight initially; people said the same thing about her. We are not all designed to be paper thin. My size two pants had space in them and I was so small that when my mom saw me she seemed concerned.

I enjoyed being called skinny. Just about everyone in America would rather be skinny than fat and Lord knows I heard more than enough how chunky I was or how I could stand to lose a few pounds. Being called skinny was a compliment. But skinny is no implication of one's physical fitness. Even at such a small size I was unfit because I was not getting the nutrients that my body needed each day for energy. I would tire easily and had to go to bed early.

What I recall most about this time in my life is being afraid to eat out or to eat in atmosphere's where I could not control the numbers. If I didn't know how many calories and fat I was eating, I was afraid to eat it. What if I eat more calories than I'm supposed to? What if I gain a pound today?

There were times when they would have lunch provided at work; I would just sit there and watch them. I would watch each of them cut into their food. I would watch the fork approach their mouths and then I would gaze as they chewed each morsel. The smells tortured me because I really wanted a bite. But the, "what if 's?" kept me from indulging.

Our lives are not to be dictated by food. Food should never be such a concern and hold so much importance in our lives that it holds us hostage. We should not be anxious about eating, instead we should seek God.

I've often thought about the fact that saying grace has become such a tradition in the homes of Christians that we don't use that time to pray for the things we really need concerning food. If you need God to help you to not overeat, ask for that as you say your grace. The Bible says that we have not because we ask not. (James 4:2)

Another thing that you can do is create boundaries that will help you not to overeat. My husband and I often order one entrée and share it. This way I am really getting one portion because the portion sizes at most restaurants are so big. This is also a great way to help your spouse practice some restraint as well and you'll be setting a good example for your children.

A friend taught me to ask for a to-go box when my food arrives. As soon as your plate comes you put half of it in the box for later. This only works if you know that you won't go in the box and eat the food you put away. You can always ask the waiter to hold it for you but if you really want it later, you may forget it if you leave it with the waiter.

In church the other day, I heard a Pastor say that his wife kills her food so that she won't eat more than she should. "That's good for her but bad for me," he said. "Bad for me because she kills my food too." What did he mean by killing her food? This is when you poor salt, sugar or some other condiment at your table all over the food once you've had enough. You are killing the food because you are making it inedible. It's dead.

This method proved to be the best method for me. When I've had enough to eat—not when I need to unbuckle my pants—but before that, I drench my food in salt. I even go as far as to put the paper from my straw in the food and any trash that I have in my purse. I don't just kill my food, I slay it!

I know some of these techniques sound absurd and even silly, but you have to be willing to do whatever it takes to live this lifestyle. This is a journey and you will go through peaks and valleys but at every point, know that God is there and when you need help, turn to Him.

What Should I Eat?

Maybe your fear is not that you will eat too much at gatherings or restaurants, maybe your anxiety comes from not knowing what foods to eat. "I just don't know what to believe, 'cause one day something is good for you and the next minute it's bad for you," a friend of mine said. She was frustrated because she had been drinking soy milk and buying everything soy and then all of a sudden there was controversy surrounding soy.

As I mentioned, Leviticus Chapter 11 describes some of the foods that were considered clean and unclean. We are told to eat creatures in the sea and ocean that have fins and scales (sorry, this excludes shellfish), which birds to avoid (hawks, owls and bats), that we should eat animals with divided hoofs that chew the cud, and that we should avoid the pig.

The Bible also makes mention of some foods very often like olives, wheat, apples, and pomegranate. Joel 1:12 says, "The vine is dried up and the fig tree is withered; the pomegranate, the palm and the apple tree—all the trees of the field—are dried up. Surely the joy of mankind is withered away." 2 Samuel 17:28 says, "...They also brought wheat and barley, flour and roasted grain, beans and lentils." They also drank goat's milk and cow's milk and ate cheese. And we know how often fish is mentioned; Jesus performed a miracle of feeding thousands with a fish dinner for one person.

Everything we need, God has provided. His word is sufficient for us to live healthy lifestyles and He makes it clear about the foods that are best for us to eat. Some will argue that those precepts are under the law and as followers of Christ, we are not under such law. That is true but I believe that if it was unclean then, it's still not the best option.

There is no need to be confused or fearful of what foods you should be eating. God's best will always be the foods that He originally ordained us to eat and that is fruits, veggies, legumes, nuts and grains (the seed bearing plants). Those are His absolute best.

The foods that we want and crave are the foods that God didn't create and probably never intended for us to eat; they are man made. Man can never outdo God, so even when we take supplements and eat meal bars; nothing comes close to the true source.

If it is processed or in a package, it's something you should only have on occasion. We were created to live long and God gave us specific foods that would help us live long lives, and sustain our organs. When we eat less of the things we need and more man made foods, we end up with diseases.

There are so many varieties of fruits and vegetables. Too often we get in a routine of eating the same foods over and over again. When I first started eating healthy the only two veggies I knew to cook were broccoli and spinach. "Honey what's for dinner?" my husband would ask on Monday. "Tilapia, rice and broccoli," I'd say. "Honey what's for dinner?" my husband would ask on Wednesday. "Turkey meatballs, sweet potatoes, and spinach," I'd say.

I eventually learned to actually read the labels in the produce section and discovered that there were so many fruits and vegetables that I'd never tried before like butternut squash, chickpeas and papaya. God has given us a rainbow of foods to eat with flavors for every taste including salty, sweet and even sour.

Here are some more ideas on fruits, legumes, grains and veggies to try.

- Artichokes
- Bock choy
- Parsnips
- Jicama
- Swiss chard
- Edamame
- Brazil Nuts
- Quinoa
- Pumpkin Seeds
- Flax seed

As far as meats go, you want to stick with leaner cuts of meat, which means meat with less fat on it. Eating leaner meats allows you to get the protein and vitamin B that you need from meat sources, while reducing the amount of fat and cholesterol found in fattier meats. I do want to caution you about processed and packaged meats. Always read the labels of these products as many contain added sodium and preservatives. Some deli meats and ground poultry can be high in fat. These are foods you should only eat occasionally.

Some great lean meats are:
- Canned tuna (In water)
- Salmon

- Skinless Chicken Breast
- Ground chicken
- Sirloin steak
- Round beef
- Chunk beef
- White, skinless meat from the turkey

Remember these staple foods: eat whole grains, lean meats, fruits, veggies, beans and nuts in abundance. Don't get caught up in the new studies and the new reports on what's good or bad. Man made items will always be controversial. You won't have to worry about that if you eat more fresh and less processed food!

❖　❖　❖　❖　❖

TINY TIP:
You think you're eating healthy when you order a salad at your local fast food restaurant, but this is not always true. The dressing that you use is where most of the fat and calories are found. Go for a fat-free, low calorie dressing!

Prayer:

Heavenly Father, I thank you for the foods you have placed here for me to eat. I thank you for properly educating me on nutrition and even showing me in your word what foods are best for me.

Lord, I desire to live a long, strong life without any sickness or disease. I believe that by faith and because I know that faith without works is dead, I ask you to help me carry out the actions of eating healthy to go along with what I am believing for.

Thank you for showing me cool, new, healthy foods to try and share these recipes with the people that I love.

Stir up excitement within me for the foods that you created just for me. You love me so much that you saw fit to provide food that would help me carry out your will. For that I am thankful and I give you praise.

In Jesus' Name,
Amen

ഔ ൙

STAY ON TRACK

It's all in what you eat,
That determines your defeat.

It's all in what you chew,
That determines your breakthrough.

It's all in what you taste,
That determines your place.

It's all up to what you choose,
At the table and in the drive thru's.

It's all up to what you choose,
If weight is what you desire to lose.

So, choose lean.
Leave the package on the shelf.
Choose fresh,
'cause that's what's best.

Stick with grains,
Eat some nuts,
To lose the gut,
Stay on track!

ഔ ൙

ഒ ☯

CHAPTER 10
ഒ ☯

The Gospel of Fitness

For physical training is of some value, but godliness has value for all things, holding promise for both the present life and the life to come.

1 Timothy 4:8

श्ली ल्क

If you flip through the pages of the dictionary and look up the word, "fitness," you might be surprised at what you discover. Webster's defines it as, "the quality or state of being fit," and it is listed as a synonym for health. Health is the synonym for fitness; they mean the same thing. "Arian, why are you pointing this out?" You might ask. It seems that we associate fitness with being skinny and looking a certain way. Being fit for many of us means being smaller or having bigger muscles. This is not what fitness is at all. Being fit means that your body is in good condition; it refers to the total condition and state of your body.

As I mentioned before I recently joined a new gym and was given a fitness assessment by one of the trainers there. He asked me what my goals were. "I really just want to be healthy," I said. He was taken aback by my comment. "Most people want to lose ten pounds or get leaner," he replied. I simply wanted to be healthy and fit and that's rare. I've been on both sides of the coin, the one who wanted just to be smaller, and then the one that wanted more muscles and a leaner body. I was the one who went from not living healthy at all to working out every day, twice a day. With that experience I've learned that the bottom line of it all is just to be healthy and that is fitness.

As simple as this may seem, it's pretty profound in our society where people are working out every day with no motivation other than to be the size they were in high school or to look like some model that they saw in a magazine. I'm in no way saying that you should not have goals. We all should have goals and strive to be better in every area of our lives. What I am saying is that your reason for living a healthy lifestyle should not be simply to look a certain way. When this is your only motivation you can become vulnerable to trying just about anything to reach that goal.

One of the items in the world of fitness that I urge you to be most cautious about is the use of supplements. There are pills and capsules for just about everything you can imagine. There are protein shakes and shots of concoctions to make you bigger or stronger or leaner. Many of these supplements can affect your body negatively if used on a long term basis. Some of them can even affect hormone levels. My husband tells of how a woman that he worked with developed a deeper voice because she took so many supplements in an effort to be leaner. You don't need these types of supplements. Just eat the foods God created and get moving.

Whether it's limiting your caloric intake to 1100 calories per day, exercising like crazy or taking oodles of supplements, none of these activities promotes good health. They promote the external benefits of good health, so while you may look good on the outside, your body is suffering internally. I mean, what's the point in spending money and wasting time on living healthy when in the end you still become sick from not taking care of your whole self?

Living in a healthy way with an external focus is what I like to call, "fleeting fitness," because it's a false form of fitness that will only last a certain amount of time. Fitness with a worldly focus will not benefit any human being for total life health. 2 Corinthians 4:18 KJV says, "While we look not at the things which are seen, but at the things which are not seen: for the things which are seen are temporal; but the things which are not seen are eternal." The things that we can see, the worldly things that we too often cherish above the heavenly pursuits, are not of importance. 1 John 2:17 NLT says, "And this world is fading away, along with everything that people crave. But anyone who does what pleases God will live forever." The craving and desire to be of a certain physique, and the practice of accomplishing that goal is temporary, it won't last.

Total Body

Focusing so much on the external elements is not the total idea of fitness. In its entirety it includes the physical; internal and external, and spiritual man. 1 Timothy 4:8 says, "For physical training is of some value, but godliness has value for all things, holding promise for both the present life and the life to come." This scripture helps us to understand that while exercising is important, the most important thing is for us to live lives that are godly and that glorify God. The Message Bible version of this scripture makes it even clearer saying, "Exercise daily in God— no spiritual flabbiness, please! Workouts in the gymnasium are useful, but a disciplined life in God is far more so, making you fit both today and forever."

Another scripture that follows this same idea is 3 John 1:2 KJV, which says, "Beloved, I wish upon all things that you may prosper and be in good health even as your soul prospereth." We focus on the prosperity connotation to this scripture but we miss out on the emphasis placed on health. It really says that as our souls prosper, so shall our health. Our souls prosper when we have a one on one personal relationship with God. It is when we see Him as our Father and commune with Him on a daily basis. It is when we read His word and make His word the final authority over our lives. It is when we seek Him first in everything that we do. As our souls prosper, so does our health.

Traditions have kept many of us from this relationship that I spoke about. Growing up and into my adulthood I thought that being a Christian meant that I went to church every Sunday, that I acted a certain way and that I didn't do certain things. I thought it meant that I could only be forgiven by God and considered righteous if I didn't do certain things. Since then I've learned that I was made righteous and that God already approves of me and you (Romans 5:19 and 2 Corinthians 5:21). Most importantly, I learned that being a Christian means that God is my Father and that I am supposed to know Him. As a child I remember writing God letters every night when I was going through some family problems. I would place the letters on my dresser believing that God would read them every night. Look at the relationship that David had with God. It was like they were best friends. David talked to God about everything; his fears, his mistakes—nothing seemed to be off limits.

The fact is, God wants us to spend time with Him. He desires to converse with us. In my time with God I discover things about myself both good and bad. I get answers to things I've been praying about or was confused about. I get filled up and doused in His goodness, leaving me with a joy that no situation that occurs that day could snatch. This is how our souls prosper.

Add the Word

One way to keep your heart pure and stay motivated to exercise and eating right is by adding the word. Tracy, my trainer would say, "Put the word in your workout." There is power in reciting God's word and calling on the name of Jesus. We discussed how adding the word can push you through the workout, but it can also keep you focused on why you are exercising in the first place.

You are doing this for God. Colossians 3:23 says, "Whatever you do, work at it with all your heart, as working for the Lord, not for men." When you exercise and when you eat the right food, that's not something you just do casually. You do it as if you were doing it for God not to be accepted; not to look like someone else.

The gospel of fitness is that fitness should be a part of every Christian's life. To believe by faith to live a long and prosperous life but not do anything yourself or act out on what you believe is almost an oxymoron. It's the same as believing God for a job but not sending in any resumes. Remember that we are taught to apply works to our faith. The things that we are believing for by faith, we should act out on.

If you are believing for a good grade on a test, your works would be to study. If you are believing for a promotion on your job, your works would be to excel in the workplace. And my dear, if you are believing God for better health or weight loss, your works would be to change the food that you eat and incorporate some type of physical activity into your lifestyle. We cannot expect God to do for us what He has empowered us to do for ourselves.

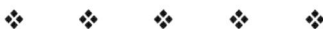

❖   ❖   ❖   ❖   ❖

TINY TIP:
Sometimes we take for granted the gift of life that we have. Too often a hospital visit is what opens our eyes to the need of change. Don't let a doctor have to tell you to change, start your healthy lifestyle today!

Prayer:

Lord, I thank you for helping me to understand your word and that taking care of my body was simply your intention for me. Thank you for the knowledge that I now have about how to take care of my body in a way that pleases you and in a way that keeps you at the focus.

Help me to carry out the principles I learned. Help me to keep first things first, understanding that this is a lifestyle; not a sprint. I know that you will provide all the grace that I need to be victorious. I know that I can do this, and now that I know what is required of me, I make the decision to take the steps needed to live healthy and whole in every area of my life.

In Jesus' Name,
Amen

ॐ ೞ

BLINDED

Walked in the gym

Barely noticed

Too thin

Wanted to be smaller

Not happy with

Herself within.

Panting and sweating

Drip

Drop

Drip

Her body collapsed.

ॐ ೞ

ജ ര

CHAPTER 11

ജ ര

You Win!

The fruit of the righteous
is a tree of life; and he that
winneth souls is wise.

Proverbs 11:30 KJV

ℰℭ ℭℛ

You're meditating on the word, renewing your mind and making fitness a lifestyle. You are walking in complete victory, and despite the struggles you face, you win! Now that you've fostered a winner's mentality about health and wellness and are aware that you are fated to win the battle because God himself is fighting for you, let's look at the bigger picture of why your health is so important to the kingdom of God.

A friend told me a story about how he was living the fast life in the music industry. He only ate take out food and drank alcohol in heavy amounts on a daily basis. He ended up in the hospital, suffering from a heart attack in his early thirties. He tells the story of how he actually died and saw a bright light, feelings of warmth, freedom, and carelessness overtook him. Apparently he lived to tell the story because he came back, but what if he hadn't? What if he had died right there in that hospital at only thirty years old? He would not have been able to carry out his purpose.

Living a healthy lifestyle is not only our reasonable service to God, but it allows us to take care of ourselves so that we can be healthy enough to fulfill the mission He gave us. We all have an assignment. Some may have a huge mission or contribution to the earth, while others may be called to their local community or even their own households. Regardless of the purpose or calling, we all have one. Proverbs 16:4 MSG says, "God made everything with a place and purpose. . ." Oprah Winfrey talked about this on her final show and she encouraged all of us to find that thing that we were called to do. It's the thing that you can do that comes natural to you and you could do it without any monetary compensation.

The Bible gives us a number of examples of people who had significant purposes, some big some small, but all were significant. Noah simply built a boat, but that boat saved mankind. Mary simply had a baby boy, but that baby boy brought light to a dark and damned world. One of my favorites is Saul, later given the name Paul, who was once a murderer of Christians was later given the mission of spreading the gospel as a prophet. His writings, now included in our Bible, are some of the most practical and easily understood scriptures, and his testimony reminds us that God can use anyone who is willing. What would we be if the people I just mentioned had not fulfilled their destiny? Whose life could you be affecting by not fulfilling yours?

One of the enemy's goals is to stop you from reaching your full potential and from discerning what you have been called to do. He does this by distracting us with the cares of life, addictions, wrong relationships, sin, and feelings of hopelessness, just to name a few. He knows that if you get to that place where God has called you to be, he can't stop you. It would be his absolute pleasure to see you eat yourself to death or settle for a lazy life on the couch. He is content with you there, but you shouldn't be. We win when we do what we were called to do, because it is in that place that others see God's glory operating inside us and are drawn to Him. It is also in that place that we find total life prosperity, as we continue in His word.

You have a reason for being here and God is depending on you to carry it out. It should encourage and motivate you towards excellence when you know that you have a reason to be here. People need you, God needs you. There is a specific function that you have on this earth that only YOU can perform. Living haphazardly and treating our bodies horribly is easy when you don't know your purpose; when you don't see the vision for your life. Once you figure it out, you begin to live on purpose and live with purpose.

Think about what you love to do. What bothers you and frustrates you? The obesity epidemic in America was something that I wanted to help solve. What solution do you have to a problem? What is your calling? Also, know that when people say you have a calling it does not mean you are called to one particular thing. We are all multifunctional because we are all called to be sons and daughters, but then we also function as moms and dads, husbands and wives. These are callings too. Additionally, you may be called to be a doctor, but also a mentor at the community center. It is fulfilling to do all those things God has planted inside you, but you can only fulfill your calling if you are healthy.

Complete the activity below:

I am passionate about these things:

_____

_____

_____

_____

I will begin carrying out my purpose in the things that I've listed by:

_____

_____

_____

_____

_____

Taking on the Mission of the Great Commission

Taking care of yourself so that you can be of sound body is also important because there are still people that need to know Jesus. If you are worried about your own health or struggling with your own addictions, it becomes difficult for you to be about the business of the Father. In addition to our career, family and volunteer roles, we are all called to spread the gospel of Jesus. Not only do we win battles, but we win souls for the Lord.

I don't say that to get you freaked out thinking that you have to go door-to-door preaching the good news. Sometimes you can minister to others simply by walking in love towards them. I've often had to say nothing on jobs, but when people see my behavior they are drawn to me. They ask questions like, "I notice that you are always smiling what's your secret?" or "Why do you workout every day?" One of the most memorable incidents happened as I sat at my desk at work. A co-worker came to me in tears and whispered, "Can we go somewhere and pray?" I was honored and befuddled all at the same time. I could only wonder what made her choose me. As we walked into an empty conference room to pray, I counted each step. "Lord, give me the words to say." I looked in every cubicle making sure everyone was in place. Prayer in corporate America was taboo. "Lord, please don't let me lose my job." Well, I didn't and we prayed and she thanked me. She continued to come to me for prayer consistently after that day.

I used these opportunities to introduce people to Christ and lead others back to Him. Many of the people that we come in contact with every day have no other connection to Christ but us. We bridge the gap. They see God through us. This is why the way we live and how we treat our bodies is so important.

You are God's envoy in the earth. Here's an example: You call your cell phone company about being overcharged $70 on your last statement. The representative responds saying, "There is nothing I can do. I think you should call back tomorrow because I am too busy to deal with this right now." Who do we usually become upset with? That's right, we get upset with the company. And we should because this person is a representative of the company and is your direct connection to the company. The relationship that unbelievers have with us is the same. When we present ourselves as Christians and act negatively towards unbelievers, it turns them off from Christianity as a whole.

At the end of the day, nothing that we do is about us. Its' always about other people. Philippians 2:3 says, "Do nothing out of selfish ambition or vain conceit, but in humility consider others better than yourselves." The greatest commands that we are given are to love God and to love our neighbor and walking in love means that we are always considering others. The latter part of 1 Corinthians 10:24 says, "Nobody should seek his own good, but the good of others." Your exercising and eating right is not for you, it's for your family and the people's lives that you are called to touch in the world. They need you to be alive and well.

You win! You win the battle and you fulfill God's purpose so that you can ultimately win souls!

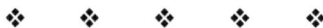

❖ ❖ ❖ ❖ ❖

TINY TIP:
Help someone else. Take your knowledge of health and fitness and add it into someone else's life that may be struggling!

Perhaps you don't know Jesus or maybe you don't know how to minister to others. Here's a prayer of salvation. I implore you to welcome the love of Christ into your heart if you haven't already.

Prayer of Salvation

Heavenly Father, your Word says that if I confess with my mouth and believe with my heart that Jesus is Lord, I shall be saved. I believe Jesus died for my sins and rose again to give me everlasting life.

Forgive me for my past, Father, and help me to begin to live a life that glorifies you from this day forward. Fill me with your spirit, Lord, and let me feel the wholeness of being your child.

I thank you for your unconditional love and for accepting me just as I am. God, I choose to never be the same again. Today I am a new creation and I choose to live a life for you.

Thank you for saving me, God.

In Jesus' Name I pray. Amen!

Scripture References:
- John 3:16
- Romans 10:9-10
- John 10:10
- Romans 5:8

ॐ ॐ

ON A MISSION

No longer fooled by

The latest gimmick,

the number on the scale or

the tag in my pants.

I won't be stopped,

Not by fast food commercials,

Or late night cravings,

Or memories from my past.

Being healthy is what I've got my eyes on,

It's much bigger than me,

Every day is a mission trip,

And I'll end it successfully.

ॐ ॐ

Review of the steps you should take:

1. Find a scripture to meditate on daily.

2. Take a multivitamin each day.

3. Start a food diary.

4. Find a support system.

5. Eliminate high fructose corn syrup from your diet (it's hidden in syrup, jelly, ketchup, even bread).

6. Don't drink calories (soda and juice), but drink water instead. 8 to 10 glasses per day.

7. Always read food labels, paying close attention to the serving size.

8. Read ingredients and always choose the products with the most natural ingredients that you can pronounce (low-fat foods and diet foods are often heavy laden with additives, sugars and preservatives).

9. Replace the breads, rice and pastas with whole grains and brown rice.

10. Use fat free and low-fat dairy products.

11. Drive by the drive thru. Prepare your own meals and make eating out an occasional thing.

12. Use agave nectar or honey as a sweetener instead of artificial sweeteners and real sugar which is high in calories.

13. Use canola and extra virgin olive oil for baking (for even healthier options substitute oil for apple sauce).

14. Eat at least five or six small meals a day. This keeps you full and helps boost your metabolism.

15. Grill or bake meats as opposed to frying.

16. Eat slowly and be aware of the food you eat.

17. Get the protein that you need each day.

18. Eat lean cuts of meat and fish such as lean turkey and salmon.

19. Eat fresh and frozen fruits and veggies; they should make up half of your plate.

20. Find an activity that you will enjoy and exercise at least 5 days a week.

21. Continue to seek God as your source of strength and keep meditating on those scriptures.

22. Never bring food into the house that tempts you.

23. Talk to other people about health and fitness.

24. Designate one day a week as a treat day, but even on that day avoid gluttony.

25. Don't be in bondage to a scale, counting calories, or pants sizes.

26. If you fall, repent (apologize to God, turn away and keep pressing ahead).

27. Warm up before exercising and stretch after.

28. Make fitness a lifestyle.

❖　❖　❖　❖　❖

CHAPTER 12

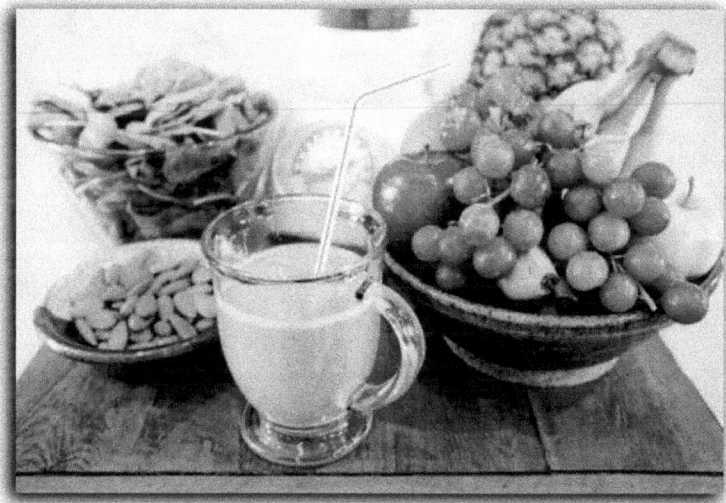

Recipes

- Breakfast -

FLUFFY PROTEIN OATMEAL

Serving Size: 1

Ingredients:

- 2 cup oatmeal
- 2 serving of protein powder (flavor of your choice)
- 2 tablespoons unsweetened applesauce

Instructions:

1. Prepare the oatmeal according to package instructions.
2. Add protein and stir.
3. Add applesauce and stir.

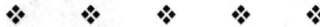

❖   ❖   ❖   ❖   ❖

When selecting a protein, please pay attention to grams of sugar, cholesterol, fat as well as the added ingredients. Pick a brand that has no artificial flavors and sweeteners.

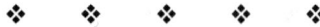

❖   ❖   ❖   ❖   ❖

MEXICAN EGGS AND TOAST

Serving Size: 1

Ingredients:

- 2 large eggs
- ½ cup spinach
- ¼ cup diced tomatoes
- 1 teaspoon chili powder
- 1 slice fat free American cheese
- 2 slices of whole grain bread
- 3 teaspoons fat free butter
- 2 teaspoons fruit spread made with real fruit (no high fructose corn syrup)

Instructions:

1. Crack one egg in frying pan after heating pan with one teaspoon butter.
2. Add egg white of the second egg and scramble.
3. Mix in spinach, tomatoes, and chili powder.
4. Break cheese into pieces and add.
5. Remove from stove.
6. Toast bread and top with butter and fruit spread.

❖   ❖   ❖   ❖   ❖

BANANA AND RAISIN BREAD

Serving Size: 1

Ingredients:

- 2 slices of cinnamon raisin Ezekiel (sprouted grain) bread
- 1 tablespoon peanut butter
- one-half chopped banana

Instructions:

1. Toast bread.
2. Spread peanut butter on each slice.
3. Top with bananas.

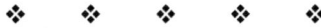

❖   ❖   ❖   ❖   ❖

When choosing a peanut butter look for one without any added ingredients. It should not have hydrogenated oils or trans-fat. Smart Balance® is an awesome brand.

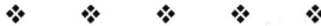

❖   ❖   ❖   ❖   ❖

BREAKFAST BURRITO

Serving Size: 2

Ingredients:

- 2 scrambled eggs
- 2 pieces of turkey bacon
- Shredded romaine lettuce
- 4 slices of tomato
- ½ cup shredded fat free or low-fat cheddar cheese
- 2 whole grain tortillas
- 1 tablespoon salsa

Instructions:

1. Scramble eggs using a low fat butter with zero trans fats (Smart Balance®)
2. Top with cheese.
3. Add ingredients (eggs, meat and veggies) into the tortilla.
4. Add salsa.

❖　❖　❖　❖　❖

FRUITY BLISS CEREAL

Ingredients:

- 1 ½ cups of Kashi® GOLEAN Crunch!® cereal
- ½ cup strawberries
- ¼ cup blueberries
- ½ small banana
- 1 cup fat free milk, almond milk or soy milk

Instructions:

1. Pour cereal.
2. Pour milk.
3. Add fruit.

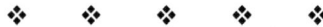

❖   ❖   ❖   ❖   ❖

Breakfast is the most important meal of the day and this one is perfect for those on the go!

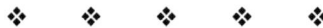

❖   ❖   ❖   ❖   ❖

- Lunch -

EVERYTHING SMOOTHIE

Serving Size: 2

Ingredients:

- 1 banana
- ½ cup spinach
- 1 orange
- ½ cup oatmeal
- 1 apple (sliced)
- ⅓ cup blueberries
- ⅓ cup strawberries
- 1 teaspoon ground flax seed
- 1 cup of water
- 1 ½ cups of frozen fruit
- 2 servings of protein powder

Instructions:

1. Put all of the ingredients into a blender and simply blend until smooth.

I love this smoothie and I often eat this for lunch. You aregetting all your servings of fruits and veggies for the day as well as some protein. It tastes delicious too!

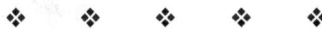

❖   ❖   ❖   ❖   ❖

Look for frozen fruit mix at your local grocer. They usually have strawberries, pineapples and mangoes mixed in.

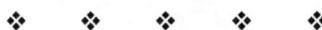

❖   ❖   ❖   ❖   ❖

BBQ TUNA SANDWICH

Serving size: 2

Ingredients:

- One can of tuna in water
- 2 tablespoons BBQ sauce
- 2 slices whole grain bread
- 4 slices of tomato (2 for each sandwich)
- 2 romaine lettuce leaves
- 2 pieces of turkey bacon (cooked)

Instructions:

1. Place tuna in a bowl.
2. Mix in the BBQ sauce.
3. Spread half of the tuna contents on one slice of bread.
4. Add lettuce, tomatoes and turkey bacon.
5. Repeat for second serving.

❖   ❖   ❖   ❖   ❖

When choosing a BBQ sauce, choose one without high fructose corn syrup.

❖   ❖   ❖   ❖   ❖

TASTE LIKE MORNING AVOCADO TURKEY SANDWICH

Serving Size: 1

Ingredients:

- ¼ cup chopped avocado
- 2 slices of whole grain bread
- 2 slices of tomato
- Shredded romaine lettuce
- 1 fried egg white
- 1 teaspoon Dijon mustard

Instructions:

1. Fry egg white in fat free butter, no trans-fats.
2. Toast bread.
3. Add Dijon to both slices.
4. Add meat and veggies.
5. Add egg white.
6. Top with avocado.

❖   ❖   ❖   ❖   ❖

TROPICAL GRILLED CHICKEN SALAD

Serving Size: 1

Ingredients:

- ½ cup shredded romaine lettuce
- ½ cup spinach
- 1 Boneless, skinless chicken breast or 1 cup prepackaged grilled chicken (Natural, no additives or preservatives)
- ½ cup mandarin oranges
- ⅓ cup slivered almonds
- 1 tablespoon dried cranberries
- 1 tablespoon Raspberry Balsamic vinaigrette
- 1 tablespoon extra-virgin olive oil
- 1 teaspoon Mrs. Dash® (salt-free seasoning blend) seasoning

Instructions:

1. Grill chicken breast using a tablespoon of extra virgin olive oil and seasoned with Mrs. Dash® seasoning original blend.
2. Place lettuce and spinach on a plate (break into pieces if needed).
3. Add grilled chicken, oranges and cranberries.
4. Top with almonds and dressing.

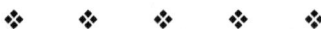

❖   ❖   ❖   ❖   ❖

MEDITERRANEAN HUMMUS WRAP

Serving Size: 1

Ingredients:

- 1 tablespoon Greek hummus
- 1 whole grain tortilla wrap
- ½ cup fresh spinach
- 2 slices of tomato
- 3 slices of turkey deli meat
- 1 tablespoon shredded fat free cheddar cheese

Instructions:

1. Spread hummus on the wrap.

2. Add meat.

3. Top with spinach, tomatoes and cheese.

❖　❖　❖　❖　❖

- D i n n e r -

SMALL TIME PIZZAS

Serving Size: 3

Ingredients:

- 4 pieces whole wheat Pita bread
- 4 tablespoons pizza sauce
- 1 ½ cup shredded fat free mozzarella cheese
- 1 cup chopped Bell pepper
- 1 cup grilled chicken (all natural)
- 1 cup fresh spinach
- ½ cup sliced zucchini

Instructions:

1. Preheat oven to 400 degrees.
2. Spread each pita slice with pizza sauce.
3. Add other toppings (meat, veggies and cheese).
4. Bake for six to ten minutes.

* Follow this delicious pizza up with a small fruit salad for dessert.

❖   ❖   ❖   ❖   ❖

THE PROTEIN SANDWICH

Serving Size: 2

Ingredients:

- 1 can of low sodium black beans
- 1 avocado
- 2 tablespoons salsa
- 1 cup chopped onion
- ½ cup chopped tomatoes
- ⅓ cup chopped cilantro
- Whole grain French bread
- 2 cups coleslaw mix

Instructions:

1. Strain black beans to remove all excess sodium.
2. Cut French bread in four parts (you'll only need two)
3. Cut each half horizontally and spread open.
4. Scoop center out from the bread.
5. Mix avocado, onions, cilantro and tomatoes in a bowl. (Be sure to smash the avocado)
6. Use a potato smasher to smash black beans.
7. Add salsa to black beans and stir.
8. Put black bean mixture on one half of the bread and avocado mixture on the other.
9. Top with coleslaw.
10. Serve chilled.

❖   ❖   ❖   ❖   ❖

SPINACH AND SALMON WRAPS

Serving Size: 2

Ingredients:

- 2 salmon fillets (6 oz.)
- 4 whole grain tortillas
- 1 ½ cup fresh spinach
- 1 packet of low sodium taco seasoning
- 2 tablespoons fat free sun dried tomato Alfredo sauce (regular fat free Alfredo is fine)
- 1 cup chopped onions
- 2 teaspoons low-fat butter

Instructions:

1. Remove skin from salmon.
2. Pan sear salmon with butter.
3. Add onions and saute.
4. Add ½ packet of taco seasoning.
5. Add spinach and stir.
6. As spinach melts down, add Alfredo sauce.
7. Place contents in tortilla wraps and serve.

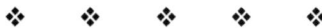

❖   ❖   ❖   ❖   ❖

SMOKIN' TURKEY TACO CHILI

Serving Size: 6

Ingredients:

- 1 lbs lean ground turkey
- 1 onion chopped
- 1 packet low sodium taco seasoning
- 1 packet Ranch dressing mix
- 1 tablespoon unsweetened cocoa powder
- 1 can of stewed tomatoes
- 1 can diced tomatoes
- 1 can of kidney beans (reduced sodium)
- 1 can of black beans (reduced sodium)
- 1 can of pinto beans (reduced sodium)
- 2 cups of salsa
- 1 avocado
- 2 chopped zucchinis
- 1 bay leaf
- 1 cup shredded low-fat or fat free cheddar cheese

Instructions:
1. Brown meat in a skillet.
2. Add beans to a soup sized pot.
3. Add veggies (onions, tomatoes and zucchini) and salsa then stir.
4. Add salsa, stewed tomatoes and diced tomatoes.
5. Add ½ packet of taco seasoning, Ranch dressing and cocoa powder.
6. Add bay leaf.
7. Let simmer for 10 minutes.
8. Serve with chopped avocado and shredded cheese.

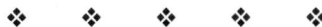

❖   ❖   ❖   ❖   ❖

WHOLE GRAIN ROTINI PASTA

Serving Size: 2

Ingredients:

- 1 cup cherry tomatoes
- 1 sliced yellow bell pepper
- 1 ½ cup broccoli
- 1 cup sliced onion
- 1 cup cleaned and sliced mushrooms
- 1 garlic clove (garlic powder is fine)
- 2 pieces of boneless, skinless chicken breast
- Whole grain rotini pasta
- 2 tablespoons extra virgin olive oil
- 2 teaspoons iodized sea sat
- 2 tablespoons Mrs. Dash® original blend

Instructions:

1. Preheat oven to 400 degrees.
2. Place tomatoes, peppers, mushrooms, onions on baking sheet or roasting pan in a single layer.
3. Sprinkle with 1 tablespoon olive oil.
4. Roast in oven for 10 minutes, stir them a bit and then place back in the oven for another 10 minutes.
5. Grill chicken using 1 tablespoon olive oil and 1 tsp salt.
6. Steam broccoli.
7. Boil pasta as instructed on packaging.
8. Mix pasta with veggies then add chicken.

❖   ❖   ❖   ❖   ❖

- Dessert -

VIRGIN APPLE PIE AND ICE CREAM

Serving Size: 2

Ingredients:

- 3 medium bananas frozen
- 1 cup fat free milk, soy or almond milk
- 3 medium gala apples (whatever you have is fine)
- 1 cup granola
- 2 teaspoons pure maple syrup
- 1 tablespoon cinnamon

Instructions:

1. Freeze bananas overnight in plastic bags.
2. Cut apples in slices.
3. Saute apples with cinnamon.
4. Add maple syrup and granola.
5. Place bananas and milk in blender and blend until it reaches a smooth creamy texture.
6. Place apples in a bowl and top with banana ice cream.

❖ ❖ ❖ ❖ ❖

CHOCOLATY FONDUE

Serving Size: 2

Ingredients:

- 1 cup of hazelnut spread
- 2 cups fresh strawberries
- 2 cups diced bananas

Instructions:

1. Place hazelnut spread in a microwave safe bowl and warm for 30 seconds.
2. Enjoy fondue by dipping strawberries and banana in hazelnut spread.

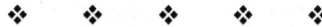

❖   ❖   ❖   ❖   ❖

PEANUT BUTTER MOCHA DESSERT SMOOTHIE

Serving Size: 1

Ingredients:

- 1 tablespoon peanut butter
- 1 tablespoon unsweetened cocoa powder
- 1 cup fat free milk, soy or almond milk
- ½ medium banana
- 1 cup of ice

Instructions:

1. Add ingredients to a blender.
2. Blend until smooth.

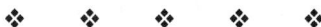

❖   ❖   ❖   ❖   ❖

OTHER DESSERT IDEAS

- When baking cakes or brownies, use unsweetened applesauce instead of oil.
- Flax seed is also a great way to get fiber and omega 3 fatty acids, so add that in too.
- Freeze your favorite yogurt flavor instead of eating ice cream.
- Make smoothie-sicles. Using either of the smoothies in this book, or your own recipe, pour smoothie into ice trays and make smoothie-sicles. Kids will LOVE this!

SNACK IDEAS

- Almonds or walnuts (only a handful)
- Carrots wrapped in turkey deli meat
- Apples dipped in peanut butter
- Kashi® Bars
- Pineapples and cottage cheese
- Fat free yogurt (without high fructose corn syrup)
- Guacamole (1 tablespoon) and tortilla chips

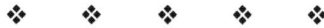

❖　❖　❖　❖　❖

TINY TIP:
Food affects the way we feel. Don't you feel sluggish after eating a huge meal loaded with fat and topped off with a dessert? That feeling usually carries over to the next morning. Why do something that makes you feel bad? Be good to your body for goodness sake!

Prayer:

Father, as I am exposed to new foods and new recipes that I have never tried before, let me be open-minded. Thank you for giving me the desire to eat healthy foods. Thank you that you will show me affordable ways to purchase the healthiest options.

I will not use the excuse of healthy food being too expensive. Instead I will find ways to do the best that I can do.

Continue to teach me to make healthier choices at the grocery store, at home and even when I am out to eat. Let my tongue and stomach crave foods that will benefit me. I thank you in advance for the weight loss that I will see as a result of my healthy eating.

In Jesus' Name,
Amen

ഇ ന്ദ

WE ALL SCREAM HAIKU POEM

Ice cream dripping down slow

Don't look! Change the channel quick

Screaming for results.

ഇ ന്ദ

හ ශ

CHAPTER 13

හ ශ

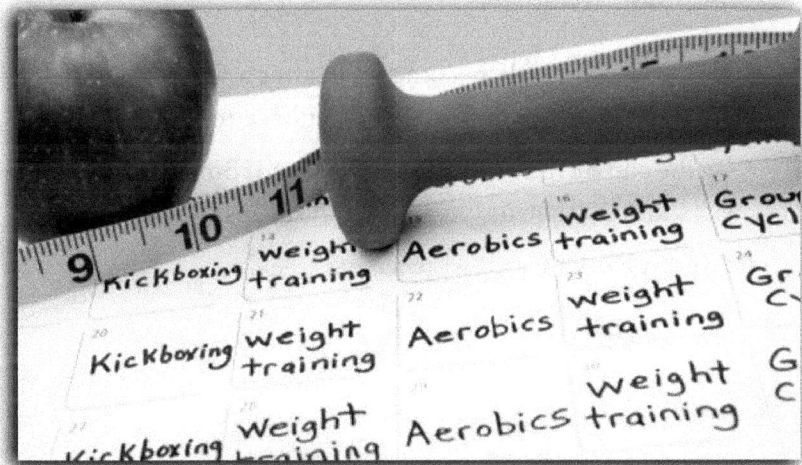

Workouts

- FROM HOME -

The Match-up

This workout is a great way to build muscle, tone and get your heart rate going. You can do it right in your bedroom or living room. It's great to do during the commercial breaks of your favorite TV show.

---

50 jumping jacks | 20 squats | 20 push-ups | 20 sit-ups

Repeat each set ten times.

- If you feel yourself become weak after a few sets, ask God for strength, take a water break and get back to it!
- By the end of this workout you will have completed 500 jumping jacks and 200 squats, push-ups and sit-ups. Way to Go!
- Do this workout at least twice per week.

Circuit Training

You will need two five pound dumbbells.

- Run in place briskly for two minutes.
- Do twelve stationary lunges; six on the right foot, then six on the left.

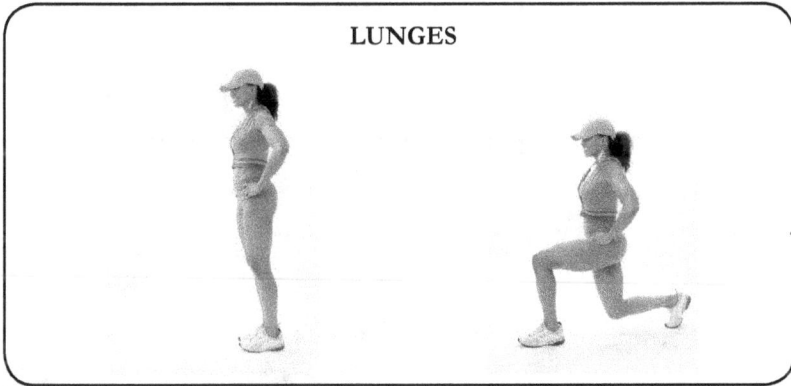

LUNGES

- Do twenty bicep curls.
- Run in place for one minute.
- Do twelve dead lifts.

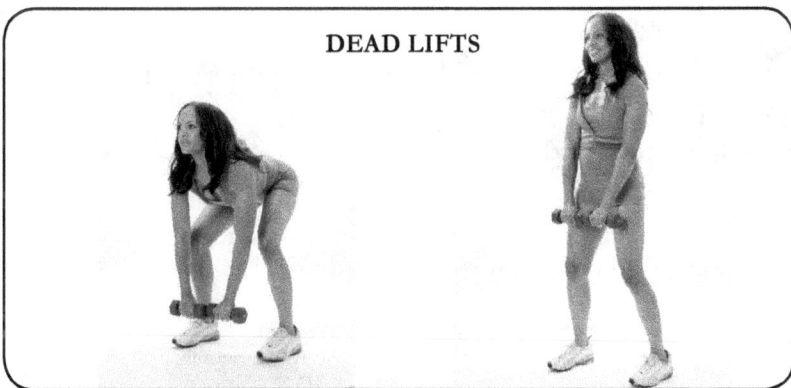

DEAD LIFTS

- Do twelve shoulder presses.
- Repeat this combination three times.
- Take breaks as needed but, no longer than 30 seconds.

Karate Yoga Mix

- Start with a warm up by running in place for one minute.
- Do high forward kicks; ten on each leg.
- Do twenty jabs; ten on each arm. Be sure to pivot your hips.
- Do twenty upper cuts; ten on each arm and pivot.

Repeat twice.

- Run in place for one minute.
- Touch your toes then jump or step back into plank.

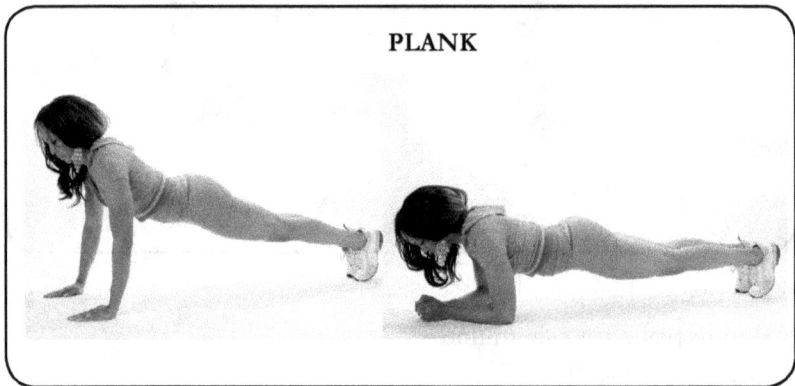

PLANK

- Go into downward dog.
- Go back into plank and lift the right leg to the sky ten times then do the left leg.
- Go into downward dog.
- Go back to plank.
- Lift each leg to your chest. Ten times on each leg.
- Back to plank.
- Jump or step back to your feet.

Repeat twice.

- GYM WORKOUTS -

CARDIO

Interval Workout

- Start on the treadmill at a walking pace of 2.5 mph at an incline of 2.5 for one minute as a warm up.

- Increase pace to 3.0. Walk at that pace for two minutes.

- Increase to a slow jog at 4.5 for one minute

- Decrease back down to a 3.0 for one minute.

- Raise incline to 6.0 and walk for two minutes.

Repeat series 'til 30 minutes. Complete strength training after cardio.

Strength Training
(Complete upper body and lower body on alternating days).

Upper Body

- 12 bicep curls.

- 12 bench presses.

- 12 tricep extensions.

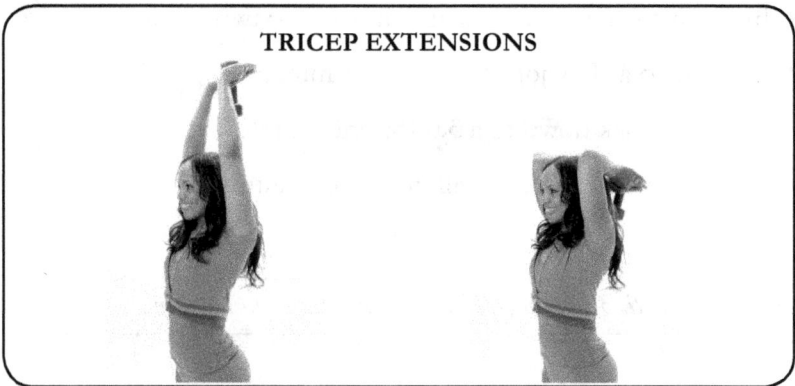

TRICEP EXTENSIONS

- 12 shoulder raises.

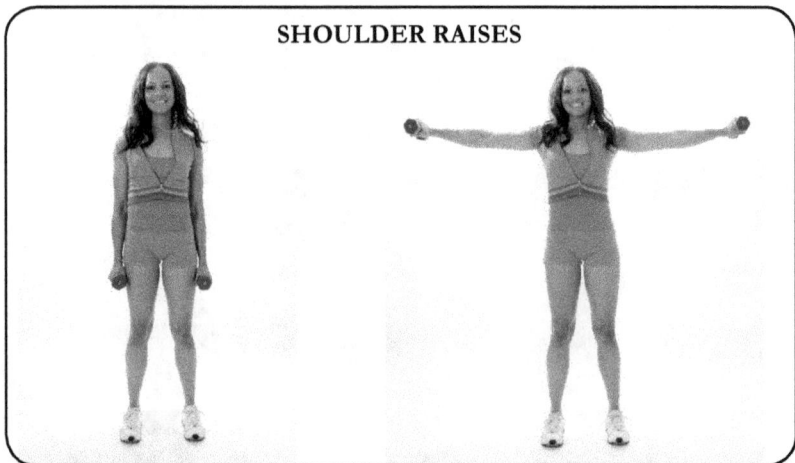

SHOULDER RAISES

Complete three times, taking a break and drinking water between each set.

Lower Body

- 12 leg extensions.
- 20 leg curls.
- 20 squats.

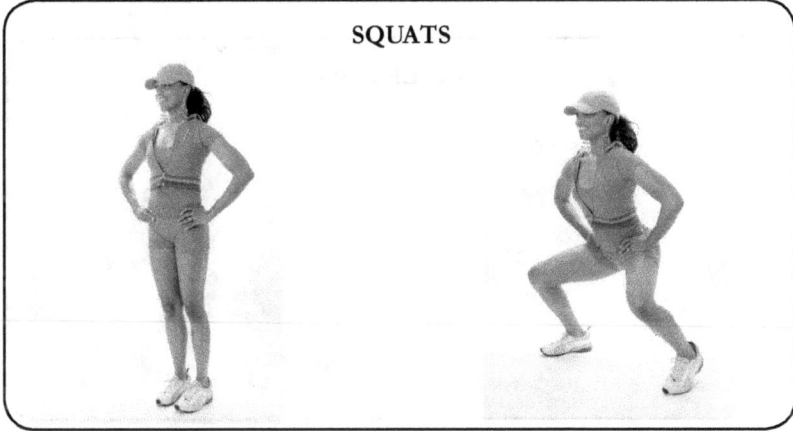

SQUATS

- 20 walking lunges holding ten pound weights in both hands.

Be sure to stretch after your workout.

Circuit Training Upper Body and Abs
(Complete upper body and lower body on alternating days.)

- Walk on the treadmill at a 2.5 mph for two minutes as a warm up.
- Increase incline to 1.5 and jog at a 5.0 for two minutes.
- Complete 20 tricep dips.

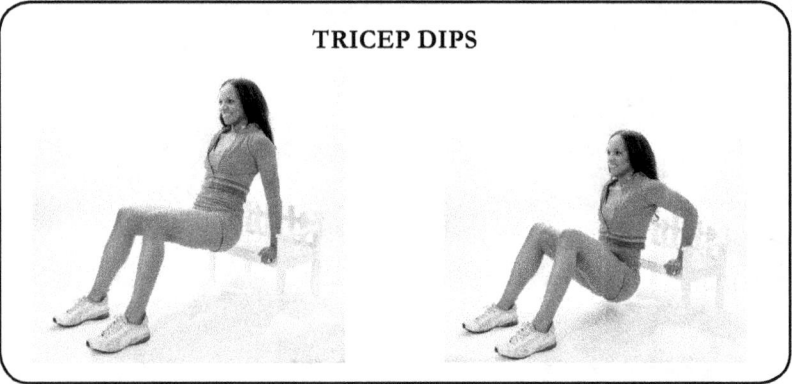

TRICEP DIPS

- Do 20 push-ups.
- Do 20 back flies.

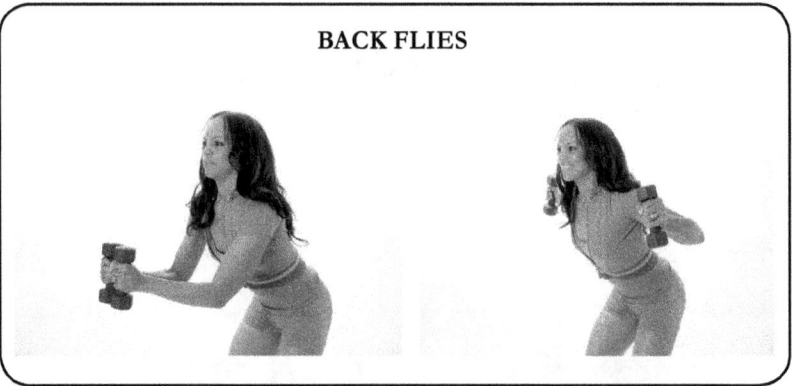

BACK FLIES

- Do 40 crunches.
- Return to treadmill and jog at a 5.0 for two minutes.
- Go back to upper body exercises.

Complete this series for 30 minutes.

Circuit Training Lower Body and Abs
(Complete upper body and lower body on alternating days.)

- Walk on the treadmill at a 2.5 mph for two minutes as a warm up.

- Increase incline to 1.5 and jog at a 5.0 for two minutes.

- Complete 20 calf raises with ten pound weights in each hand.

- Do 40 fire hydrants; 20 on each leg.

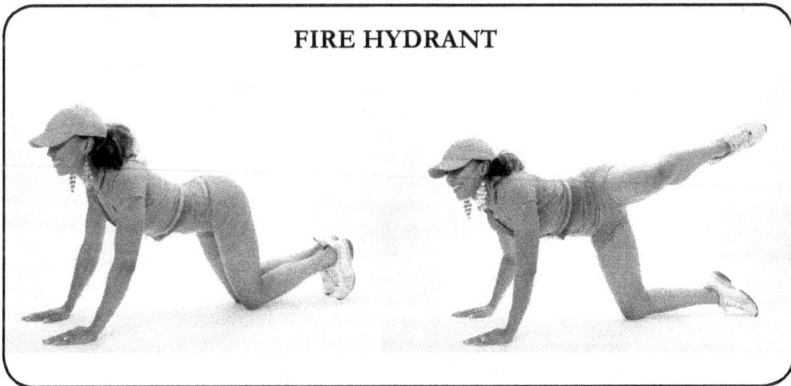

FIRE HYDRANT

- Do 20 leg presses.

- Do 40 sit-ups.

- Return to treadmill and jog at a 5.0 for two minutes.

- Go back to lower body exercises.

Complete this series for 30 minutes.

*Do upper and lower body on alternating days.

Be sure to stretch after your workout.

Other Ideas for Activity

- Go for a 30 minute a walk. Run or jog for 2 minutes, then walk for 5 minutes. Repeat till 30 minutes.

- Run up and down a flight of stairs ten times and do 20 push-ups each time you make it to the bottom.

- Wear ankle weights while vacuuming the floor and then do squats as you wash dishes.

- Wear a weight vest as you take a 30 minute power walk.

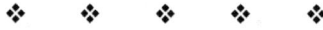

TINY TIP:
Persistence is the key to seeing results! Don't be discouraged after a week of exercise. Keep going; you'll be pleased with the end result!

Prayer:

Father, thank you that I have mobility in my body and limbs to even be able to exercise. Thank you for the continuous desire to honor you with my body through activity. Speak to me as I workout. Strengthen me to be able to carry out each exercise.

I thank you that I will desire to exercise and that it will be enjoyable for me. Give me ideas for other exercises I can incorporate into each day.

In Jesus' Name,
Amen

ॐ ॐ

I CAN MAKE IT

How many more sets?

We're not finished yet?

I'm tired,

I need a break.

This is so tough,

I've had enough.

What time is it?

I need a rest.

Breathe. Push. Pause.

I'm working for a cause,

I can make it. Whew!

I'm...I'm…done.

ॐ ॐ

Bonus Section:

Not only do you want to make fitness a part of your life, but you also want to make your overall health a priority. Honoring God with your body means taking care of each and every part. This means brushing your teeth and flossing every day. Did you know that root canals have been linked to heart disease? It should also be noted that the foods that we eat also affect our tooth health, so by eating some things less often we get a double benefit.

Getting enough sleep every night is also paramount to your health. Sleep is often something that is overlooked, but it is the self-rejuvenating and healing process that God gave our bodies. Your muscles repair as you sleep.

Finally, going in for regular check-ups should be marked on our calendars each year. I know that there are 40 million of us without healthcare, but there are free clinics around the country that might be right around your neighborhood. Contact your local health department for more information.

As you go on your journey of health and wellness, remember that everything you need lies within you. You have the Holy Spirit there to lead and guide you. Trust, lean and depend on God every step of the way. Don't be fooled by the temporal lusts of wanting to look a certain way. Remember, the ultimate goal is not to reach a number or size, but to be whole and healthy, thereby making you able to carry out your divine purpose on this Earth. I believe in you and I know that this is only the beginning to all the greatness that God has in store for you!

BIBLIOGRAPHY

1. Hill, James and Rena Wing. "The National Weight Control Registry." *The Permanente Journal.* (2003):36. http://xnet.kp.org/permanentejournal/sum03/registry.html

2. Crow, Sarah. "10 Secrets to Easier Labor." *Parents.com.* http://www.parents.com/pregnancy/giving-birth/labor-and-delivery/10-secrets-to-an-easier-labor/

3. "Hospital Support for Breastfeeding: Preventing Obesity Begins in Hospitals." *Centers for Disease Control,* CDC.gov. http://www.cdc.gov/vitalsigns/BreastFeeding/

4. "Creatine," *Medline Plus. U.S. National Library of Medicine. National Institutes of Health,* nlm.nih.gov http://www.nlm.nih.gov/medlineplus/druginfo/natural/873.html

5. Salahi, Lara. "Weight Loss Drugs: Public Citizen Calls for Ban on Alli, Xenical." *ABCNews.com* April 14, 2011. http://abcnews.go.com/Health/w_DietAndFitness/weight-loss-drugs- consumer-watchdog-calls-ban-alli/story?id=13376523

6. Schlosser, Eric. *Fast Food Nation: The Dark Side of the All-American Meal,* New York, NY: Harper Collins, 2009.

7. Parker, Hilary "A Sweet Problem: Princeton Researchers find that High-fructose Corn Syrup Prompts Considerably More Weight Gain." Princeton University, Mar 22, 2010. *Princeton.edu.* http://www.princeton.edu/main/news/archive/S26/91/22K07/

8. "Transfat," *American Heart Association*, Heart.org. http://www.heart.org/HEARTORG/GettingHealthy/FatsAndOils/Fats101/Trans-Fats_UCM_301120_Article.jsp

9. Conis, Elena. "Saccharin's Mostly Sweet Following," *Los Angeles Times*. Dec 27, 2010. Latimes.com http://articles.latimes.com/2010/dec/27/health/la-he-nutrition-lab-saccharin-20101227

10. "Sodium: How to Tame your Salt Habit Now." *Mayo Clinic*, mayoclinic.com http://www.mayoclinic.com/health/sodium/NU00284

ॐ ଓଃ

ABOUT THE AUTHOR

Arian T. Moore is a fitness nutrition coach, inspirational speaker and writer. She has been interviewed on radio and television shows for her fitness and wellness expertise. She has over ten years of experience in the field of communications after working in radio, television and print. Arian is currently an editor for Faith and Fitness Magazine.

ॐ ଓଃ

www.ingramcontent.com/pod-product-compliance
Lightning Source LLC
Chambersburg PA
CBHW070805280326
41934CB00012B/3059